THE GRASSROOTS LOBBYING HANDBOOK

THE GRASSROOTS LOBBYING HANDBOOK

EMPOWERING NURSES
THROUGH
LEGISLATIVE AND POLITICAL
ACTION

Christine M. deVries
Marjorie W. Vanderbilt

The authors are staff members of the Department of Governmental Affairs of the American Nurses Association. Between them, they have over thirty years experience in the legislative arena, and have brought to this publication their combined knowledge and experience from working on Capitol Hill, directing grassroots legislative efforts, and lobbying Congress and the executive branch.

The American Nurses Association is the full-service professional organization representing the nation's two million registered nurses through its 53 constituent associations. ANA advances the nursing profession by fostering high standards of nursing practice, promoting the economic and general welfare of nurses in the workplace, projecting a positive and realistic view of nursing, and working with the Congress and regulatory agencies on issues affecting nurses and the public.

Library of Congress Cataloging-in-Publication Data
    1. Nurses– United States– Political activity– Handbooks, manuals, etc.
2. Lobbying– United States– Handbooks, manuals, etc.
I. Vanderbilt, Marjorie W. II. Title.
    [DNLM: 1. Lobbying. 2. Nurses– United States. 3. Power (Psychology)
WY 16 D514g]
RT86.5.D48   1992
324' .4' 024613–dc20

ISBN 1-55810-078-4

Published by American Nurses Association
600 Maryland Avenue, SW
Suite 100 West
Washington, DC 20024-2571

GR-4 7.5M 3/93

"GOVERNMENT IS A TRUST
AND THE OFFICERS OF THE GOVERNMENT ARE TRUSTEES;
AND BOTH THE TRUST AND THE TRUSTEES
ARE CREATED FOR THE BENEFIT
OF THE PEOPLE."

Henry Clay
Speech at Ashland, Kentucky
March, 1829

TABLE OF CONTENTS

FIGURES

HOW NURSES CAN EFFECT CHANGE

INTRODUCTION

Knowledge is the key to power. With the information contained in this book, nurses will have the power to use the legislative, regulatory, and political processes to effect change in our society — specifically, to strengthen the health care system and the practice of nursing.

The First Amendment to the United States Constitution (1791) states that,

> "Congress shall make no law . . . abridging the freedom of speech, or of the press; or the right of the people peaceably to assemble, and to petition the Government for a redress of grievances."

In other words, a key component of our democratic government is the right to lobby policy makers to ensure that our interests and concerns are heard; it is the freedom to ask questions, make suggestions, and debate results. Lobbying is an essential part of the political process. It provides competing interests and views with an opportunity to be heard, and it provides legislators with information on which to base their decisions.

In the following pages, the basics of lobbying — from the definition of the term to the relationship between legislative and political action — will be explained. This book is intended to teach skills — the skills needed to develop a legislative agenda and to have that agenda enacted into law. Although the focus is on the federal system of government, it is important to note that these skills can be utilized in any situation, including initiatives in state and local governments.

Writing a letter to a policy maker may mean your representative in Congress, but it can also mean your representative in the state assembly, your representative on your county council, your governor, your mayor, your town council representative, or the president of the United States. The essential elements in crafting a letter to persuade a policy maker to adopt a particular point of view are the same regardless of to whom that letter is sent.

Nurses can play a special role in the legislative and political arenas. Nursing's legislative and regulatory agenda encompasses four basic goals:

1. maintain control of practice;
2. have an impact on health care policy;
3. advocate on behalf of the client; and,
4. institute workplace reforms.

The skills used in the practice of nursing in a health care setting are not unlike the skills needed to develop a grassroots lobbying campaign. Organization, interaction with people, and the development of strategies are key elements in influencing the legislative process. We hope this publication inspires you to action.

CHAPTER I

WHAT IS LOBBYING?

Lobbying is the art of persuasion — attempting to convince a legislator, a government official, the head of an agency, or a state official to comply with a request — whether it is convincing them to support your position on an issue or to follow a particular course of action.

Anyone can be a lobbyist, and everyone should lobby on issues that concern them. Most people have lobbied at some time, although they may not realize it. Have you ever tried to convince an elected official, a community official, or your boss to take a stand on a specific issue? If the answer is yes, you have experience as a lobbyist.

Although lobbying can be conceptualized in very broad terms, this guide will focus on lobbying as the act of influencing a government entity (whether it be Congress, a state legislature, or a city council) to acheive specific legislative or regulatory change.

At the turn of the century, lobbyists were portrayed as shady characters, sitting in smoke-filled rooms or hanging out in the halls of Congress. Later, they were portrayed as stereotypical short, fat, balding men emerging from limousines to pass out wads of money to greedy politicians.

Over the years, as the lobbying profession grew in size, diversity, and sophistication, much of the stigma associated with the lobbying profession disappeared. Past images no longer accurately portray the role of the lobbyist in today's political arena. Corporations, associations, labor unions, civil rights groups, foreign nations, citizen groups, farmers, and other special interest groups employ paid lobbyists in Washington, DC, and have organized volunteers around the country to carry out coordinated lobbying campaigns. Although their methods may vary, these groups share a common purpose — to exert pressure on Congress to obtain a desired goal.

From abortion to farm aid to maternal and child health to veterans' housing, every issue before Congress attracts the attention of competing interest groups. Those groups, and their lobbyists have a powerful voice in determining the outcome of legislation. Counted among those who lobby are not only traditional career lobbyists, but, also, grassroots coalitions that obtain power from their numbers and the fact that — although their headquarters may be located in Washington, DC, or another large city — they have members who reside in the home district or state of a legislator (e.g., the National Organization for Women [NOW], the National Rifle Association [NRA]).

The most visible lobbyists are those who work full-time in Washington, DC, or in a state capital and are employed by an association, corporation, public relations firm, or other interest group. Many of these lobbyists are individuals who once held jobs on congressional staffs or in federal agencies. Former Members of Congress also frequently find jobs as lobbyists or as so-called "rainmakers" in lobbying and public relations firms, because they are able to attract clients who want to develop contacts on Capitol Hill and in the White House. It is estimated that there are approximately 20,000 lobbyists in the Washington, DC area. More than 600 law and public relations firms and more than 11,000 corporations, associations, and interest groups in the United States and abroad have retained Washington, DC representation.

Constituents have an even more important role in the legislative process. Constituent pressure manifests itself in millions of letters, postcards, telephone calls, and visits to Members of Congress each year, either asking for assistance or supporting or opposing legislation before the House and Senate. This grassroots lobbying is a very effective tool because Members want to be responsive to their constituents; thus, they tend to treat grassroots lobbying with great respect, and often use it as a barometer of what the most popular course of action might be.

CHAPTER II

METHODS OF LOBBYING

"THERE IS NO POLITICAL
GAIN IN SILENCE AND
SUBMISSION."

Ms. Sidney Abbott
American writer

There are many different methods to achieve one's goals in the legislative arena. Prior to World War II, bribery was a very prevalent *legal* form of lobbying. Money traded hands on the steps of the U.S. Capitol as payment for a certain vote on a specific bill. Although this type of lobbying has been outlawed for several decades, some may argue that cases such as ABSCAM and the so-called "Keating Five" savings and loan scandal demonstrate that the use of political favors in getting votes is still the technique used by some lobbyists. Today, however, such cases are the exception rather than the rule.

The most common form of lobbying is the face-to-face approach. With this method, the contact is primary. The process involves working with individual Members to shape legislation. As a lobbyist, you can provide invaluable information on specific issues. A lobbyist (paid or volunteer) meets directly with a Member of Congress or a member of his or her staff to request a desired action, or an individual or association testifies at a hearing. Although this type of lobbying most often is associated with a paid lobbyist, volunteer members of an association or private citizens can and should utilize face-to-face lobbying. The most effective strategy is for both the paid lobbyist and the volunteer or grassroots constituent to coordinate their calls or visits to influence a legislator.

The second and most effective method of lobbying is *grassroots lobbying*. No entity with a paid lobbyist is successful unless there is a committed constituency backing up that lobbyist. In a grassroots mobilization effort, an association (regardless of its size or budget) can demonstrate the power of its constituency through action on the state and local level. The commitment must be present, but any organizational membership which organizes for direct action can be successful. Members of Congress *want* to hear from their constituents, and they will listen.

There are several different methods of grassroots lobbying. The first is letter writing campaigns — on a specific issue or piece of legislation — addressed directly to Members. The second is educational campaigns designed to mobilize public opinion and, thus, have an impact on the opinions of Members. For example, the senior citizen community became outraged by the imposition of a new Medicare supplemental premium (or surtax) for catastrophic health-care benefits that many felt would duplicate benefits they already had. They wrote to their Members in large numbers, and they went to the media and the public with their outrage. As a result, Congress succumbed to the pressure and only sixteen months after passing the Medicare Catastrophic Insurance Act, voted to repeal it.

The third method used to influence public policy is through political contributions and fund-raising. A *political action committee* (PAC) — often an arm of a corporation, association, or labor union — provides campaign support either to persuade a policy maker to back a certain program, or, more often, to ensure that a policy maker who supports the organization's goals remains in office. Political involvement through PAC activities greatly enhances an individual's access to a policy maker and is a complementary aspect of lobbying. It is essential that those who work with Congress support their friends, and contributions are a tangible means of expressing one's loyalty as well as one's political opinions.

In the following pages, each of these lobbying methods will be described in detail. Topics included for discussion are the development of a legislative agenda; legislative research tools; the processes of the federal government; the development of key lobbying contacts; congressional committees; lobbying strategies and the utilization of coalitions; PACs, and the role of the media in your lobbying efforts.

Remember, lobbyists are anyone and everyone — people with diverse political agendas focusing on the arenas where decisions are made and policy is implemented.

CHAPTER III

GRASSROOTS LOBBYING

DEVELOPING A LEGISLATIVE AGENDA

One of the many missions of the American Nurses Association (ANA) is to advance the legislative agenda of professional nursing. To accomplish this, ANA brings together lobbyists and political-education staff members to coordinate activities with individual nurses and with the state nurses associations (SNAs) to promote its legislative agenda on Capitol Hill. Each of the cogs in this perfectly greased wheel works with the others to have a significant impact on the proceedings of the Congress.

This process is a proactive one. Nurses propose legislation, persuade a Member of Congress to introduce it, build a public relations campaign around the legislation, and get the bill passed and signed into law. Once a bill is enacted, ANA lobbyists, in conjunction with state nurses associations (SNAs), lobby the federal agency responsible for promulgating the regulations that implement the law to ensure that the intent of Congress is realized.

It is the responsibility of the governing members of an association to approve the legislative agenda, but it is the primary function of the organization's staff to advance it. Depending upon the size and type of group, the procedural steps involved in developing an agenda will vary. In a large organization, such as ANA, many people are involved in approving an agenda. In a small group, consensus can be reached more easily.

In designing a legislative agenda, it is important to make sure that the proposals are politically viable. Policy makers will not take a legislative agenda seriously if it contains unattainable goals. For example, although free health care for all people is a worthy goal, neither structures nor funds exist at the present time to meet such a goal. Legislators are more willing to discuss how to improve access to the health care system for under-served populations.

Congress no longer has the ability to enact legislation without regard to its budgetary impact. Because unlimited sources of funds do not exist anymore, it is beneficial to include a funding mechanism in any proposal.

At the outset, a group needs a rationale for developing an agenda. Are you a community association whose aim is to lobby the city council for a stoplight at a major intersection? Your agenda is limited to one issue. Are you a state association whose aim is to lobby the state legislature to modify the tax laws in your state? If that is the case, your agenda may be very broad-based. You may want to identify what specific aspects of the tax laws you need to address.

After you have developed your goals or legislative agenda, you must decide if you are going to formulate an approval process. In a large group, it is useful to appoint a board of decision makers and grant them final authority for approving your agenda. Another method is to select individuals who are knowledgeable about legislation and appoint a committee on legislation to approve the agenda. This approval process lets the public know that your legislative agenda is formally approved by a body of experts. It also eliminates the time and energy that can be wasted trying to reach a consensus among too many people on too many details.

The next step is to develop (a) position paper(s) on your legislative goals. The legislative agenda of an organization is meaningless unless it is communicated effectively. Producing the position paper shows that you are knowledgeable on the subject and professionally organized. You may understand the facts and have persuasive arguments, but these are to no avail unless the people you are trying to persuade understand them. After you have discussed and approved the basic goals in your legislative agenda, it is necessary to write a brief summary of each issue. To write your position paper(s), you must be very familiar with your position and your arguments. Presenting your arguments concisely and in order of importance is helpful.

Be familiar with the opposition's arguments and craft your position very carefully. Research the issue as much as possible. Keep your paper to one page. Avoid the temptation to expand it. If you cannot organize your thoughts in one page, you will not be able to articulate your position to legislators in a few minutes. Limiting your position paper to one page does not preclude your leaving a ten-page analysis of the issue with your legislator. However, the first page of that analysis should be the executive summary or position paper on your legislative agenda, with attached copies of supporting analysis, documents, articles, and statistics.

To maintain a professional look, develop a format for your position paper. If your budget permits, print on paper with the organization's logo beside the name of your group: this adds to your credibility. Although the specific format is not important, it is important to maintain a consistent format — e.g., "Issue Briefs" — when drafting papers on different issues. The goal statement is often listed first, e.g., "The position of the California State Nurses Association on health care reform is . . . ."

A subhead devoted to "Background" is useful to state in a few sentences the history of the issue, quickly educating the group you are trying to influence. Assume that your target group has little or no understanding of the issue and state your information in simple language. Another subhead entitled, "Position," should provide a clear statement of the position of your group. This section should include a short statement explaining your identity, your membership numbers (if important), and an exact statement of your position. For example, "The Mississippi Health Care Coalition, comprised of 200 health-care professional associations in the State of Mississippi, supports legislative efforts to impose a surtax on tobacco products."

A final subsection entitled, "Rationale," can be where you present your case in two to three paragraphs. Include only the most compelling reasons for supporting your position. The reasons should be worded persuasively and may refer to supporting material or statistics. For example, "Government statistics demonstrate that applying a tax on tobacco products decreases the sale of those products by 50 percent, and results in a 30 percent decrease in the incidence of lung cancer."

Be prepared. You need to know the points that will be raised in opposition to your position, who will make them, and the reasons for the opposition of those individuals or groups. Anticipating objections can work to your advantage. First, it gives you the opportunity to brief your Member of Congress on where the trouble is; and, second, it provides you with the opportunity to prepare your counter-arguments before the opposition attacks.

Always remember to identify your group and provide a contact name, address, and telephone number in your position paper. It is safe to assume that your legislative agenda will be reproduced and disseminated beyond what you have done and people should be able to contact you after they have received your materials.

Finally, limit your legislative agenda. Although it is tempting to take on the world, you may be able to handle effectively only a small portion of your agenda at a time. Although some organizations will convene to accomplish a single legislative goal, many other groups have diverse agendas. Decide on your priorities and take on only what you can handle.

With a legislative agenda in hand, you are now prepared to begin to lobby on your issues.

FIGURE 1

AMERICAN NURSES ASSOCIATION LEGISLATIVE AGENDA

The ANA is a federation made up of 53 constituent state nurses associations (SNAs). A discussion of the procedures governing the development of ANA's legislative agenda follows.

Input by a SNA member on any topic of interest is referred to ANA staff who, in turn, refer the matter to the appropriate structural unit within the association. In this particular case, it is the Committee on Legislation (a committee of the Board of Directors of ANA) which considers proposed legislative positions. The committee formally solicits input from the appropriate congresses and other governing bodies of the association on the potential impact of the proposal in terms of nursing practice and economics. Once this information is procured, it is the responsibility of the committee — in conjunction with ANA's Department of Governmental Affairs and ANA's Department of Policy Development — to develop a policy statement that is in accord with the legislative and policy agenda of the association. The committee on legislation has the authority to approve any policy presented by a governing body, with ratification required by the full ANA Board of Directors for assimilation into the association's legislative agenda.

The legislative agenda of the association is, in part, derived from the association's strategic plan. For example, Goal VI of the association's strategic plan is, "To achieve effective control of the environment in which nursing is practiced and services offered." From this broad goal, specific legislative goals are drawn. Goal VI is the source of many legislative and regulatory goals, e.g., "Protecting employment rights of employees in health care facilities" and, "Supporting access to legislation that provides reimbursement for nurses in advanced practice." From these legislative and regulatory goals, ANA's Department of Governmental Affairs identifies specific bills in Congress and regulations in federal agencies that are important to ANA's and the SNAs' legislative missions.

The culmination of the previously stated broad goals was the passage of the Civil Rights Act of 1991 and the Nursing Rural Incentive Act of 1990, both identified as priorities for the association. All of this information is included in the publication, *ANA's Legislative and Regulatory Initiatives,* along with accompanying positions papers on each identified legislative and regulatory issue. This publication is an invaluable resource for educating Members of Congress and the public on nursing's legislative agenda.

RESEARCHING LEGISLATIVE AND REGULATORY ISSUES: DOING YOUR HOMEWORK

Once you have developed your legislative agenda, the next step is working for its implementation. A successful lobbying campaign requires a well-thought out strategy that includes identifying whom to lobby, the critical junctures at which to influence the legislative and regulatory processes, and effective lobbying techniques.

Prior to formulating this strategy, however, it is necessary to develop some expertise on the issue involved. It is not necessary to get a Ph.D. in the legislative subject area, however, because you can always arrange a meeting between a technical expert and the policy maker if the situation should require it. Instead, you should equip yourself with supporting data, personal anecdotes, and an analysis of the impact of your legislative proposal before you talk to your legislator.

In today's legislative and regulatory environment, where the number of issues seems to multiply daily, the ability to provide pertinent information is crucial. It is your job as a lobbyist to provide the information to the Member of Congress. That material should be concise, precise, and persuasive.

Eventually, you want to be recognized by your legislator as a vital source of information on certain issues, someone whom the legislator calls upon for information and advice. You will become a valuable asset by helping him or her answer constituents' questions, and by providing witnesses at public hearings, assisting in the drafting of specific language in legislative and regulatory proposals, and providing opinions on other proposals. It is important for nurses to be identified as health care experts and to participate in discussions on the reform of the health care system at all levels of government.

Members are interested in the impact that legislation may have on their congressional districts or their states. State assembly representatives are interested in a proposal's impact on a specific neighborhood. Demonstrating the local impact of a proposal is an effective lobbying strategy. For example, in arguing for the need for direct reimbursement for advanced practice nurses, it is beneficial to show how this process would enhance access to health care for unserved and underserved populations. To justify a child care center, demonstrate how such a center would benefit the community's workplaces.

In gathering your information, include both concrete data and personal stories. Be able to document all your information. Do not try to fake it. If you do not know the answer to a question, say so, then indicate that you will obtain the requested information and get back to the legislator.

Remember: no one has all the answers to all the questions. Above all, *never misrepresent the facts*. If you get caught, your credibility with the legislator will be lost forever. Honesty is always the best policy.

USING STATISTICS EFFECTIVELY

- PUT THE NUMBERS IN HUMAN TERMS.

  "Cutting existing health care costs by $1 billion will mean every man, woman, and child in this country will be forced to forego some necessary preventive services."

- SIMPLIFY THE NUMBERS.

  "Americans spend $666 billion on health care every year. This can be broken down to:
  > $1.8 billion every day
  > $76 million every hour
  > $1.3 million every minute
  > $21,000 every second."

- AVOID PERCENTAGES.

  Use "two out of three" rather than 64 percent.

- USE NUMBERS SPARINGLY.

  Choose two or three meaningful statistics and be sure to identify their significance.

  "There are three key figures on this chart. They are . . . ."

- USE FEDERAL, STATE, AND LOCAL NUMBERS.

  "There are approximately 37 million uninsured Americans, 1 million of whom live in this state, and 10,000 of whom reside in this county."

- KNOW YOUR NUMBERS.

- BE PREPARED TO CITE YOUR SOURCE.

RESOURCES TO UTILIZE IN RESEARCHING ISSUES

To gather as much information as possible to prepare for your lobbying efforts, it is important to know where to find it. A wealth of information exists for those documenting positions on policy issues. Some information is easy to obtain and is free; it is simply a matter of putting your name on a mailing list. Other resources are very costly and will be utilized only by organizations with significant lobbying budgets. Often, several groups will get together and share the cost of a publication.

The recent emergence of sophisticated computer programs has created services that can provide enormous amounts of information via databases available on-line to subscribers. Some services provide information on federal legislation and regulations (e.g. "Legis-late"), and are updated on a daily basis to assist lobbyists, as well as Members of Congress and their staffs. Lists of bills introduced, congressional hearings scheduled, reports issued on a bill, and profiles of Members are included. Similar services exist for legislation introduced in state legislatures (e.g. "State-Net").

USING PERSONAL STORIES EFFECTIVELY

- FIND PEOPLE WHO RESIDE IN A SPECIFIC CONGRESSIONAL DISTRICT OR AREA IN ORDER TO INFLUENCE A SPECIFIC POLICY MAKER'S DECISION.

  For example, since the chairman of the House Energy and Commerce Committee's Subcommittee on Health and the Environment is from Los Angeles, it would be useful to locate, in the chairman's home area, a family that has no health insurance and is confronting a serious medical problem.

- KEEP THE STORIES SIMPLE.

  It is not necessary to explain every detail, but it is critical to give the policy maker enough information so he or she understands how the situation evolved.

- BE SPECIFIC ABOUT WHAT YOU WANT.

  Explain how a proposed bill would either: 1) improve the situation or correct a problem; or, 2) harm the status quo.

- TELL THE STORY IN STRONG, DECLARATIVE SENTENCES.

  "Providing treatment centers for drug-addicted pregnant women would decrease the number of boarder babies in this country."

- USE THE STORY TO STRESS THE IMPORTANCE OF THE ISSUE.

  "The tragedy of this family illustrates why health care reform must dominate Congress' agenda."

- USE THE STORY TO MAKE A REQUEST.

  "We urge you to consider immediately the passage of legislation to increase funding for nurse education programs in order to address the nursing shortage in our country today."

- DON'T LIE.

If you are a member of a national association, that association is one of your most valuable resources. For example, if you are a nurse who belongs to a SNA, both that SNA and the staff of the ANA can provide you with information on legislation and regulations. In addition, associations often publish legislative newsletters and updates that describe legislative and regulatory initiatives of importance to their membership. One such publication, *Capital Update,* is published by the ANA Department of Governmental Affairs (Please see inside back page for subscription information).

Legislative Resources

Tracking the status of current legislative issues often is perceived as a formidable task, requiring an in-depth knowledge of the issue, a vast library of costly publications, and an intimate understanding of the workings of the federal government. This is not necessarily true. While the researcher may be aided by access to documents and an understanding of the legislative process, it is possible to follow an issue using a variety of resources that are readily available.

Bills, Committee Reports, Conference Reports, Public Laws

Legislative documents (bills, committee reports, conference reports, and public laws) are available from the House and the Senate document rooms. One copy each of six different documents may be requested in writing daily from the Senate Document Room, and one copy each of twelve different items may be requested in writing daily from the House Document Room. You should enclose a self-addressed, gummed label for return mailing and send your request to:

SENATE DOCUMENT ROOM	**HOUSE DOCUMENT ROOM**
Room SHB-04	Room B18
Hart Senate Office Building	Ford House Office Building
Washington, DC 20510	Washington, DC 20515
(202) 224-7860	(202) 225-3456

The House and Senate each maintain document rooms to distribute their own legislation. They serve Members' offices, committees, and the public. Each document room maintains files of the other chamber's legislation, but as a rule will only distribute copies to Members' offices or to committee staff. The public must go directly to the House Document Room to obtain House items and to the Senate Document Room for Senate items. Public laws are available through both document rooms. The Senate Document Room does not accept phone orders. The telephone number listed is for information purposes only. The House Document Room does accept phone orders.

Legislative Information System (LEGIS)

When you do not know specific details about a bill, you may telephone the *legislative information system* (known as *LEGIS*), a computerized information bank, at (202) 225-1772. The operators can search for legislation by subject, title, sponsoring/co-sponsoring Member's name, bill number, etc. You can receive an update on any House or Senate bill including date of introduction, sponsors and co-sponsors, dates of committee and subcommittee hearings, and the status of the bill. Remember, the legislation must have been introduced in the House and/or the Senate for the operators to be able to respond to your inquiry. The system cannot track "legislation" that *may be* introduced. However, you can ask whether any measures on a certain subject have been introduced. You will be asked to identify your organization when you call.

House Calendar

The House Calendar provides complete and accurate legislative histories of all House and Senate legislation once it has been reported by a committee. It also has information on conference committee action and new public laws. The Monday edition contains a subject index. The calendar is updated each day the House is in session and is available free of charge from the House

Document Room or by subscription from the Superintendent of Documents, Government Printing Office (GPO), 710 North Capitol Street, NW, Washington, DC 20401, (202) 783-3238. Visa and MasterCard are accepted.

Daily Congressional Activities

Both the Democrats and the Republicans in the House and Senate provide recorded messages of the proceedings on the floor of each chamber every day they are in session. This includes information on floor debate, scheduling, and voting. The telephone numbers for these recorded messages are:

SENATE	(202) 224-8541	(Democratic)
	(202) 224-8601	(Republican)
HOUSE	(202) 225-7400	(Democratic)
	(202) 225-7430	(Republican)

White House Records/Presidential Signature

The Office of the Executive Clerk of the White House can provide information on when a bill was signed or vetoed, and give the dates of presidential messages, executive orders, and other official presidential actions. This office can be reached at (202) 456-2226. Refer to the bill number when calling. As bills are signed by the president, public law (PL) numbers are assigned to them, in chronological order, by the Office of the Federal Register, Presidential Documents Legislative Division at (202) 523-5230.

Congressional Record

The *Congressional Record* is published by the GPO each day that one or both houses are in session, except when House and Senate sessions are very brief, in which case two or more consecutive issues are printed together.

The *Record* is the primary source of information on what happens on the floors of the House and the Senate. It provides a substantially verbatim account of all debate in the House and Senate and records how each Member voted on all recorded votes.

Senators and representatives are allowed to edit their remarks before they are printed in the *Record*, correcting grammatical mistakes and even changing words spoken in the heat of debate. Speeches not given on the floor may be included, although both the House and Senate have tightened the rules governing *inserting remarks*, as this process is known. The full texts of bills and other documents, never read aloud on the floor in their entirety, often are printed in the *Record*.

The *Record* contains the following four sections:

- *Proceedings of the House and Senate.* These are edited accounts of floor debate and other action taken in each chamber. Prior to March, 1978, there was no way to ascertain whether a Member had actually delivered his or her remarks or, instead, had had them inserted in the *Record*. Since then, inserted remarks are noted in the House proceedings by a different typeface (from a standard to an italicized style), and in the Senate by black dots, or bullets. If a Member reads only a few words from a speech or article, it will appear in the *Record* as if it had been delivered in its entirety.

Since 1979, time cues have marked House floor proceedings in the *Record* to show the approximate time a debate or discussion occurred. Senate proceedings have no indication of time.

- *Extension of Remarks.* This is material not read in whole or in part on the House or Senate floor, but, instead, merely inserted in the *Record.* It can include such extraneous material as speeches given outside Congress, or copies of newspaper articles, editorials, or letters. Senators may add such material to the body of the *Record;* Members of the House must place it in the *Extension of Remarks* section.

- *Daily Digest.* This section summarizes House and Senate floor action for the day, and provides a listing of subcommittee, committee, and conference committee meetings held, including summaries of the witnesses who testified. It also notes bills reported, conference reports filed, and the times and dates of the next meetings of subcommittees, committees, and the full House and Senate. The week's last issue of the *Digest* lists the program for the coming week, including legislation scheduled for floor action (if it has been announced), and all committee and sub-committee meetings.

- An *Index* to the *Record* is published twice a month and can be used to locate bills by subject.

About 20,000 copies of the *Record* are published daily. In Fiscal Year 1990, this cost $17.9 million. An annual subscription costs approximately $1,200 a year. (Until 1970, a subscription cost $1.50 month.) Single copies of a specific issue of the *Record* or an annual subscription may be ordered from the Superintendent of Documents (see address, *House Calendar*, p. 13).

Each senator is entitled to 40 free copies and each representative to 25 free copies of the *Record* for distribution to constituents. If you are interested in receiving a subscription in this manner, you should write to your senators and/or representative. Although their allotments of subscriptions may be exhausted at the time you write, you can ask to be placed on a waiting list. These subscriptions often change hands rapidly.

Digest of Public General Bills and Resolutions

This *Digest* lists all bills and resolutions, as introduced in Congress, in numerical order, with a detailed description of each piece of legislation. Enacted bills also are listed, showing subject and author. Published twice during each session of Congress, the *Digest* is available from the Superintendent of Documents.

Committee Calendars

Committee calendars usually list committee and subcommittee membership, committee publications, and legislation referred to the committee, along with any action taken on it. Frequently, these calendars also list the legislative jurisdiction of the committee and its subcommittees and the committee rules. Committee jurisdictions and rules also are often published in a separate *committee print*. You may obtain committee calendars directly from each committee's document clerk.

Committee Hearings and Schedules

The *Daily Digest* in the back of each issue of the *Record* lists hearings for the next day. The last edition each week lists publicly announced hearings for the following week.

In addition, inquiries can be made directly to the committee and subcommittee staffs.

Committee Prints and Hearing Records

To obtain a free copy of a committee print or hearing record, send a self-addressed label to the publications clerk of the committee that issued the document. Generally, hearing records are available two months after the end of the hearings.

In addition, all House and Senate hearings and prints can be purchased through the GPO. When ordering by mail, include all pertinent information. Payments may be made in cash, check, money order, credit card (Visa, MasterCard) and through GPO deposit accounts. Prices given for each document include postage and handling. No tax is charged.

For questions and information on congressional hearings and prints (e.g., prices, if a document is available, etc.), call (202) 275-3238.

Legislative History

The chronology of a law can be traced by obtaining a copy of the law from the House or Senate document room or from the GPO. At the end of each law as printed is a summary of all action taken on it prior to its enactment, including dates of House and Senate passage and *Congressional Record* citations.

Congressional Quarterly Weekly Reports

Congressional Quarterly Weekly Reports are published by Congressional Quarterly, Inc., 1414 22nd Street, NW, Washington, DC 20037. The *Reports* are published weekly, with special supplements and an annual *Almanac*.

These are weekly compilations of congressional action and developments. There are sections on committee and floor action, a table indicating the status of major legislation, and charts showing recorded votes in both chambers. It also includes articles on current legislative issues.

The annual *Congressional Quarterly Almanac* is a comprehensive review of the legislative session. A subscription to the *Weekly Reports* and *Almanac* is approximately $1,300 a year. To subscribe, call (202) 887-8621 or (202) 887-8500.

Congressional Monitor

The *Congressional Monitor* is published by Congressional Quarterly, Inc., Monday through Friday when Congress is in session.

This is a daily summary of congressional activities, including all scheduled committee and subcommittee hearings (with a list of witnesses, if available) and meetings, as well as conference committee meetings. Also included is appropriations legislation status, a list of legislation to be considered on the House and Senate floors that week, and a summary of committee and floor action for the previous day.

The *Monitor* is available by subscription for about $1,300 annually. Subscribers also receive access to a "hotline" question-and-answer service, a 24-hour tape recording of the day's highlights on Capitol Hill, and *Congress in Print* — a weekly listing of committee publications. To subscribe, call (202) 887-6279.

National Journal

The *National Journal* is published weekly by National Journal, Inc., 1730 M St., NW, Suite 1100, Washington, DC 20036.

This periodical contains reports on various current public policy issues and provides background information and analysis of the issues currently under consideration by Congress and the executive branch. For subscription information call (202) 857-1448 or (800) 424-2921. The annual subscription rate is approximately $775. Public and academic library rates, as well as student and faculty rates, are lower.

Compilation of Presidential Documents

The *Compilation of Presidential Documents* — with quarterly, semi-annual, and annual indexes — is published weekly by the GPO. This periodical is the source of information on the dates when the president signed or vetoed legislation. In addition, it provides transcripts of presidential messages to Congress, executive orders, and speeches and other materials released by the White House.

Many of the publications cited above can be found in local public libraries. The publications of the federal government can usually be found in libraries designated as federal depository libraries. GPO bookstores in more than 25 cities throughout the United States can be found by consulting a local telephone directory under the listing, "U.S. Government."

Another valuable source of information is your Member of Congress who is elected to office to serve you. You should always keep a record of your Member's Washington and district office(s) telephone numbers. Your Member will send you copies of bills, reports, or public laws at your request. Many also have newsletters that they send out to their constituents on a regular basis, explaining their initiatives and votes in Congress. To receive these newsletters, call or write your Member and request that your name be placed on the appropriate mailing list.

Some Members' caucuses and task forces publish their own newsletters. For example, the Congressional Caucus on Women's Issues publishes a monthly twelve-page newsletter which updates readers on legislation affecting women. You can receive this newsletter free of charge if your representative is a Member of the Congressional Caucus for Women's Issues. Other available resources include many of the support services of the Congress. With the advent of C-SPAN and C-SPAN II, many people can watch the proceedings of the House and Senate in their own homes.

If you are unable to spend hours in front of the television, however, there are telephone numbers which will provide you with up-to-the-minute information on proceedings on the House and Senate floors. The staffs of the House and Senate cloak rooms (the antechambers off the floors of the House and Senate) will answer your questions regarding whether a bill has come up for floor consideration that day or which amendment is being considered. In addition, there are tape recordings (the *cloak room tapes*) providing pre-recorded information on daily House and Senate floor activities. These tapes are updated on a regular basis when Congress is in session.

Switchboard in the Capitol

The office of any Member of the House or Senate — as well as any committee or subcommittee — can be reached by calling (202) 225-3121 or (202) 224-3121 and asking to be connected to the specific office.

Federal/Regulatory Resources

Code of Federal Regulations

The *Code of Federal Regulations* (*CFR*) is published by the GPO. Each year, as of January 1, April 1, July 1, and October 1, a separate one-quarter of the titles is revised.

The *CFR* codifies final regulations which are legally binding and which have appeared previously in the *Federal Register*. They are arranged by subject in 50 titles (approximately 190 volumes). With the annual revision incorporating new regulations and dropping those superseded, the *CFR* reflects regulations in effect at the time of printing. Several indexes and tables accompany the set.

Federal Register

The *Federal Register* is published by the GPO on Monday through Friday, except holidays.

The *Federal Register* serves as the official announcement of regulations and legal notices issued by federal agencies. These include presidential proclamations and executive orders; proposed and final federal agency regulations; documents required to be published by an act of Congress; and other federal agency

FIGURE 3

IMPORTANT CONGRESSIONAL TELEPHONE NUMBERS

(202) AREA CODE

Capitol Switchboard	225-3121 or 224-3121	Operator Assistance
Clerk of the House	225-7000	Committee membership lists
Senate Daily Digest	224-2658	Availability of bills
House Daily Digest	225-2868	Availability of bills
Senate Democratic Cloakroom	224-8541	Tape of floor action and scheduling information
Senate Republican Cloakroom	224-8601	Tape of floor action and scheduling information
House Democratic Cloakroom	225-7400	Updated tape of current House floor action
House Republican Cloakroom	225-7430	Updated tape of current House floor action
Legislative Information	225-1772	House: status of bills
Senate Enrolling Clerk	224-6250	Whether a bill has been sent to the White House
House Enrolling Clerk	225-5848	Whether a bill has been sent to the White House
Executive Clerk	224-4341	Status of treaties and nominations
Senate Majority Leader	224-5556	
Senate Majority Whip	224-2158	
Senate Minority Leader	224-3135	
Senate Minority Whip	224-2708	
House Speaker	225-5604	
House Majority Leader	225-0100	
House Majority Whip	225-3130	
House Minority Leader	225-0600	
House Minority Whip	225-0197	
Speaker's Room	225-2204	Scheduling information

documents of public interest. It also functions as an update to the *CFR*. Daily and monthly indexes and an accompanying publication, *List of CFR Sections Affected,* assist in its use.

As is the case with legislation, there are times when more regulatory activity information is required than is available in printed materials. Oftentimes, too, assistance is needed in using the printed sources. For those instances, the Finding Aids Office at the *Federal Register* can identify the location and date of recent items appearing in the *Federal Register* and can assist in using the *CFR*. Its number is (202) 523-5227.

The Public Information Office can send single copies of the *Federal Register* until the supply is exhausted. It also can supply up to ten pages of photocopies for a nominal cost. The office can be reached at (202) 523-5240.

White House Records

The office of the Executive Clerk at the White House can provide information on the dates that executive orders and presidential proclamations appeared in the *Federal Register*. The telephone number is (202) 456-2226.

WHERE TO LOBBY: PROCESSES OF THE FEDERAL GOVERNMENT

The next step in the development of a successful lobbying campaign is to understand how our government works. To influence legislation, you should understand how a bill becomes law and how the legislative branch interacts with the other branches of government. Of critical importance in these processes is the congressional leadership — the Members, elected by their colleagues, who shepherd bills through the legislative system and serve as the chief advocates for the legislative agendas of their parties.

With knowledge of the important actors and processes, you can focus on key points in the legislative process and on key players in the Congress, and mount an effective lobby campaign.

FIGURE 4

STRUCTURE OF THE FEDERAL GOVERNMENT

LEGISLATIVE BRANCH	EXECUTIVE BRANCH	JUDICIAL BRANCH
CONGRESS: US HOUSE OF REPRESENTATIVES/ US SENATE	**WHITE HOUSE** President	**SUPREME COURT** Courts of Appeal
General Accounting Office	Vice President	District Courts
Congressional Budget Office	Cabinet	
Library of Congress	Federal Departments and Agencies	
- Congressional Research Service	Office of Management and Budget	
Office of Technology Assessment	Council of Economic Advisors	
	National Security Council	

BASIC STRUCTURE OF THE FEDERAL GOVERNMENT

The United States government at the federal level consists of three branches: the executive, the judicial, and the legislative.

The executive branch consists of the office of the president, the office of the vice president, and the federal departments and agencies. Its primary duties include recommending legislation, administering laws, and signing or vetoing legislation. Every year, generally in late January, the president delivers a State of the Union address to a joint session of Congress, presenting a blueprint setting the course of action for current executive branch policy.

The executive branch implements laws through the regulatory process. Regulations are printed in the *Federal Register,* usually with a comment period for input by the general public. The regulatory process is important because it is possible for regulations to be issued that do not follow the congressional intent of the law. In such cases, it is necessary to lobby the federal agencies to change the regulations and, failing that, to go back to Congress to clarify the law's intent.

The judicial branch of the federal government is the court system. The courts' primary responsibilities are interpreting laws and changing existing law within their jurisdictions.

The Supreme Court is the highest court in the nation and can, essentially, establish its own agenda. Because of this, the Supreme Court can insert itself directly into the debate on issues when it decides to influence public policy. The checks and balances of our government, however, give Congress the power to supersede an unpopular Supreme Court decision through enactment of new legislation.

In the recent past, legislators have been more conservative than the courts and hence, the courts preceded Congress in effecting social change. For example, prior to the passage of the 1964 Civil

Rights Act, civil rights cases were taken through the court system and won. That trend is no longer apparent with the recent appointments of conservative justices to the Supreme Court. Today, we find the Congress to be the agent of social change and progress, repeatedly attempting to pass laws to overturn Supreme Court rulings in cases limiting the interpretation of laws.

The court system is divided into two parts: the federal and the state court systems. The federal court system includes district courts and twelve circuit courts of appeal. The state court system includes trial courts, intermediate appellate courts, and state supreme courts. Generally, federal courts interpret laws on education, employment, violations of the Constitution, and crimes that take place on federal property. State courts address family law, most crimes, and the interpretation of state laws.

The third branch of government is the Congress, a *bicameral* (two-chamber) legislature comprised of the House of Representatives and the Senate. The chief function of Congress is to make laws. In addition, the Senate has the function of approving the ratification of treaties and nominations by the president. The Senate has the sole authority to approve federal circuit court and Supreme Court nominations. In the matter of impeachments, the House of Representatives presents the charges (a function similar to that of a grand jury) and the Senate sits as a court to try the impeachment.

The House and Senate meet in joint session on January 6, following a presidential election, to count the electoral votes. If no candidate receives a majority of the total electoral votes, the House of Representatives chooses the president from among the three candidates having the largest number of popular votes, and the Senate chooses the vice president from the two candidates having the largest number of votes for that office.

The heart of the government is the legislative branch with its responsibility for listening and reacting to the needs of the people. A term of Congress lasts two years — e.g., 1993 is the first session of the 103rd Congress, and 1994 the second session. Members of Congress hold their seats because they are elected by "the people back home," who expect their interests to be represented at the national level. Two senators are elected from each state, each representing the entire state. Senators serve a six-year term; every two years, one-third of the Senate is up for re-election. Recently, the District of Columbia elected a *shadow senator,* but this official has no voting and only limited participatory power in the Senate.

Representation in the House of Representatives is determined by the population of each state. A House Member represents a district of approximately 500,000 to 600,000 people. Every ten years, House membership is reapportioned based on the results of the decennial census and the redrawing of congressional districts. There are 435 Members of the House. Because each representative serves a two-year term, the entire House is up for re-election every two years. Having to face re-election every two years (House) or six years

(Senate) ensures that Members keep the needs and interests of their constituents in mind when considering legislation.

The unique constitutional responsibility of the House is to originate legislation that deals with the spending of money and the raising of revenue.

HOW A BILL BECOMES A LAW

"Congress has been in session nearly two months, and only three bills have passed and become laws. None of them is of national import."

— The Washington Post
February 21, 1892

Approximately 10,000 pieces of legislation are introduced over the two-year life of each Congress and fewer than 1,000 are signed into law during that period (see Figure 5). For example, in the 101st Congress, there were approximately 9,200 bills and resolutions introduced, but only 650 of those became public laws. Of the bills introduced, 1,187 — or almost 12 percent — were health-related. During the 102nd Congress, approximately 11,700 bills and resolutions were introduced, but only 590 of those became public laws.

During a congressional session, any senator or representative may introduce legislation. The proposal may call for a change in existing law or the creation of a new program. There are unlimited

---

FIGURE 5   HOW MANY BILLS BECOME LAW?

PERCENTAGE OF BILLS INTRODUCED THAT BECOME LAW

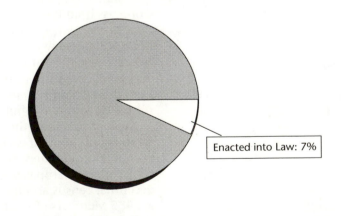

Enacted into Law: 7%

The Grassroots Lobbying Handbook

sources of ideas for legislation. The executive branch may request that a bill be introduced in response to a presidential or federal agency initiative. In such a case, the chairman/chairwoman of the committee to which the bill would be referred generally will introduce the measure. If he or she does not support the proposal, he or she may introduce it "on behalf of" or "by request" of the administration. Private groups, organizations, or individuals also can initiate legislation by asking a senator or representative to introduce a bill.

The length of the legislative process varies tremendously. Some bills may be enacted during the course of one Congress, while others may take years of debate, re-introduction, and redrafting before being enacted. Emergency legislation can be drafted, introduced, and acted upon in a matter of hours. Other issues become timely because public interest has focused on them — child care, AIDS, homelessness, and crime, for instance. Most bills introduced, however, never see congressional action and ultimately die. Because Congress is bicameral, all bills must pass both the House and the Senate before being signed into law by the president.

Once a bill has been introduced in either house, it is referred to the standing committee, in that chamber, that has jurisdiction over the issue with which the legislation is concerned. If the bill addresses several issues, it may be referred to several committees.

In both the House and Senate, it is a common practice for the sponsor of a bill to send a *Dear Colleague* letter to other Members, explaining the purpose of the bill and asking them to co-sponsor it. This practice increases support and gives other Members and the public an opportunity to see who is lining up behind a bill. An agreement to co-sponsor is not binding, however. Members may request to have their names withdrawn or may decide to oppose a bill when it gets to the floor.

There is no limit on the number of Members who can cosponsor a bill. Original co-sponsors are listed on the front of the bill after the sponsor's name. However, Members may add their names as co-sponsors anytime after a bill has been introduced, although their names will not show up on the printed text of the bill. Their co-sponsorship is cited in the *Congressional Record*. Although bills are not reprinted to list co-sponsors added after the date of introduction, a current and complete list may be obtained by calling the Legislative Status Office at (202) 225-1772.

Members of Congress often will respond to constituent support for a bill by co-sponsoring it. This not only permits the Member to express support for an issue before it is ever voted on, but it also helps to advance the prospects for the bill by broadening its base of support. Bipartisan co-sponsorship increases the prospects of a bill being acted upon, as does co-sponsorship by Members of the committee to which the bill has been referred.

FIGURE 6   **THE PATH OF LEGISLATION**

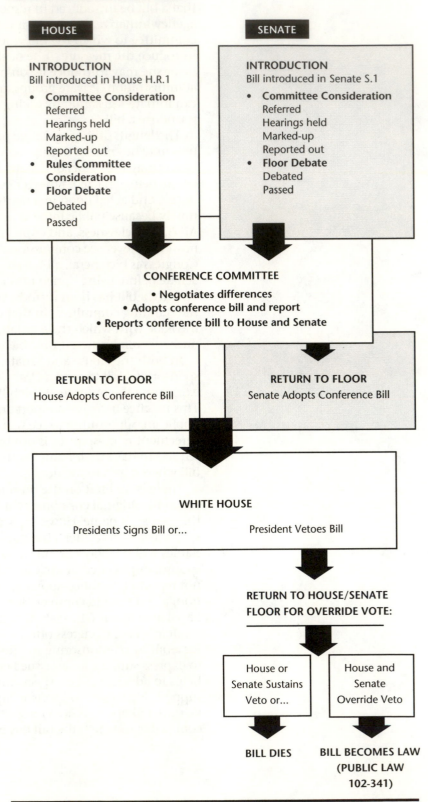

Committee Action

In most circumstances, for legislation to see full committee action, it must be considered first on the subcommittee level. The committee chairman/chairwoman usually assigns a bill to a subcommittee. Most subcommittees have specific jurisdictions, so this decision is not arbitrary.

It is essential that there be sufficient interest in a bill for a subcommittee chairman/chairwoman to schedule hearings. That interest can be generated in a number of ways, including writing letters to the subcommittee and committee Members, endorsing the legislation, and requesting a hearing on it.

The discretionary power of the chairman/chairwoman can be seen in his or her scheduling of hearings and mark-up sessions. If the chairman/chairwoman decides to hold a hearing, often witnesses from his or her own congressional district or state are welcome and sought out. This can be an excellent opportunity to advance your cause. In addition, witnesses at hearings may include officials from the executive branch, other Members of Congress, and interested groups and individuals. Verbatim transcripts of hearings are recorded and printed for congressional and public use.

Depending on the subject matter of legislation being considered, hearings may last a few hours, several days, or even weeks or months. There are times the chairman/chairwoman will limit the type and number of individuals and organizations who may testify. This is done either to expedite the subcommittee's or committee's deliberations or to emphasize one particular point of view. Those individuals and groups who are not able to testify can submit written statements to be included in the hearing record.

There are times when hearings are needed to educate Members on specific issues. For example, in 1991 and 1992, hearings were held in numerous subcommittees and committees on the issue of health care reform. These hearings focused on specific pieces of legislation, and on broader issues, such as international health-care systems and the economic analyses behind the rising costs of health care in this country. This provided Members with valuable insight into the the health care system, as well as the views of and proposals advocated by interested groups and individuals. Members then had adequate background information to put together a major legislative initiative.

After all the testimony is gathered, the subcommittee, with the help of the staff, begins the *mark-up* process, actually marking up the legislation, writing sections, then changing them, rearranging them, adding and deleting language. The real crafting of legislation begins, as amendments to change the bill are offered by subcommittee Members. Amendments agreed to in subcommittee are incorporated into the bill, which is then approved and voted out of the subcommittee and referred to the full committee.

At the full committee level, additional hearings may be held and more amendments offered during additional mark-up sessions. If, for example, an interest group failed in its efforts to have an amendment adopted in subcommittee, it can try again in full committee. When the committee completes its deliberations, the bill is *ordered reported* or *reported out* to the full House or Senate for a vote.

Floor Action

In the Senate, after a bill has been approved by the full committee, the bill's sponsors work with the leadership to schedule floor consideration. The Senate leadership considers Senate committees' and individual senators' meeting schedules, speaking engagements, and travel plans in an effort to arrange for the Senate's business to be transacted in accordance with the membership's wishes. Unlike the House, both germane and non-germane amendments may be offered to almost any bill on the Senate floor at any time. Debate time is generally unlimited in the Senate, but not in the House. A *filibuster* — a delaying tactic where one or more senators speak until and if sixty senators vote to cut off discussion — may occur in the Senate, but not in the House.

Since the House is much larger than the Senate — with 435 Members for the former, 100 Members in the latter — it has a more elaborate set of rules. When a bill is voted out of committee in the House, it is placed on a *legislative calendar* (schedule), a roster of legislation ready for floor consideration. Reported bills are placed on the calendar in the order they were reported, but they are not brought up for floor consideration in chronological order. In fact, many bills are never brought up for consideration and, consequently, die on the calendar.

In the House, the Rules Committee has jurisdiction over the flow of bills to the House floor. Sponsors of bills and Members of the committee(s) with jurisdiction appear before the Rules Committee — which is closely allied with the House leadership — to request a *rule* governing when and how their bills will be considered by the full House. The committee determines how long the debate will be, who will control the debate time, how many, if any, floor amendments will be considered, and when the votes on final passage of the bill will occur.

A bill may be amended during floor debate. However, since Members rely heavily upon committee decisions and expertise, amendments on the floor need considerable support to win approval.

Once a bill is passed, it is sent to the other chamber where the entire legislative process is repeated.

Conference Committees

If a bill has passed both the House and the Senate in the same form, it is immediately *enrolled* and delivered to the president. If one chamber has adopted non-controversial amendments to the bill, the other chamber will generally concur by *unanimous consent*. If, however, the House- and Senate-passed versions differ substantially, the differences must be resolved by a *conference committee*.

The conference committee is usually comprised of senior Members of the committee(s) that handled the bill *(conferees)*. House and Senate conferees are appointed, respectively, by the Speaker of the House and the presiding officer of the Senate, both of whom rely heavily on the advice of the chairmen/chairwomen and ranking minority Members of the committees that considered the bill. The House Democratic Caucus' rules require that the Democrat/Republican ratio in the full House be reflected in the selection of House Members to each conference committee. The size of the House and Senate delegations of a conference committee may vary. However, since each chamber has only one vote during conference, a large representation does not give one chamber a voting advantage over the other chamber's conferees.

Entirely new provisions cannot be added to a bill during a conference. During their deliberations, conferees are limited to consideration of the matters in disagreement between the two versions of the bill. The conference committee may accept in full, accept in part, or reject each of those provisions.

At this stage of the legislative process, constituents, political action committees (PACs), lobbyists, and the White House have one more opportunity to influence the final language of a bill through personal visits, letters, telegrams, and phone calls — not only to Members of the conference committee, but, also, to other Members who may be able to influence the conferees. Immediately before and during the meetings of a conference committee, it is not unusual for conferees to be contacted *(lobbied)* by their non-conferee colleagues whose constituents have an interest in the legislation under consideration.

The conference may last a few hours, several weeks, or many months. The conference committee reconciles the differences between the two versions of the legislation and reports to the full House and Senate the conference/compromise bill and the accompanying conference report. This conference version must be approved by both the House and Senate and generally cannot be amended on the floor. Passage by a simple majority of both houses means that the bill is ready for the president's signature.

If, however, no agreement is reached by the conferees, or either the House or Senate does not accept the conference agreement, the bill dies. If a bill fails to pass both houses, it is possible for a Member to re-introduce it in a slightly modified form. It is assigned a new bill number and must go through the entire legislative process again.

Enrollment

After a bill has been passed by both the House and the Senate in identical form, it is sent to the enrolling clerk of the chamber in which the bill originated. The enrolled bill is then printed on parchment paper. When the bill has been certified as correct by the Secretary of the Senate or the Clerk of the House (depending which chamber the bill originated in) it is signed first (no matter whether it originated in the House or Senate) by the Speaker of the House and then by the president of the Senate. Then it is sent to the White House for presidential action.

There is usually a short delay between final congressional passage and the time that an enrolled bill is delivered to the White House. The White House Records Office ([202] 456-2226) can tell you whether the bill has been received at the White House and whether it has been acted upon by the president.

Presidential Action

The Constitution provides that once an enrolled bill is delivered to the White House, the president has ten days (excluding Sundays) to act. The president's options follow.

1. *approve the legislation* — the bill becomes law the day it is signed unless otherwise specified in the act.

2. *approve the legislation by doing nothing* — when Congress is in session, the bill becomes law if the president takes no action within ten days. This occurs when he or she believes it is unnecessary or politically unwise to sign the bill, or if he or she is uncertain about its constitutionality.

3. *pocket veto* — the bill dies when the president fails to sign it and does not register his or her objections. This can occur only when legislation is passed near or at the end of a session of Congress and adjournment occurs before the president has had the ten-day period in which to return the bill to Congress for further consideration. In this instance, the bill will not automatically become law. Therefore, if the president objects to a measure passed at or near the close of a Congress, he or she may "pocket" the bill until after adjournment, thus allowing it to die.

4. *veto* — when — prior to the expiration of the ten-day period — the president does not want a bill to become law, he or she can return it to the chamber of Congress in which it originated, without his or her signature and with a message stating his or her objections. Then, Congress can attempt to override the president's veto and enact the bill. If the veto is overridden by separate two-thirds (of each body's membership) votes in the House and in the Senate, the legislation becomes law. Otherwise, it is dead.

When bills are passed and signed, or passed over a veto, they are assigned a public law number. Public law numbers run in sequence starting at the beginning of each Congress. For example, Public Law 102-6 would be the sixth public law enacted in the 102nd Congress and Public Law 102-124 would be the 124th public law enacted in the 102nd Congress.

THE BUDGET PROCESS

In early February of each year, the president submits a proposed federal budget to Congress. This document represents a year of work by agency officials, who channel their budget requests up to the cabinet level, and, from there, through the Office of Management and Budget (OMB), which brings the requests into line with the president's programs. Congress then receives this final work on proposed spending levels.

Frequently, funds for certain projects are spread over a number of years. For example, if Congress approved funding for a five-year rural-health demonstration project at a total cost of $50 million, this would appear in the budget as $50 million in *budget authority*

FIGURE 7

BUDGET CHART:
SAMPLE RURAL HEALTH DEMONSTRATION PROJECT

($ millions)

	1ST YEAR	2ND YEAR	3RD YEAR	4TH YEAR	5TH YEAR
Budget Authority	$ 50	$ 0	$ 0	$ 0	$ 0
Outlays	$ 10	$ 10	$ 10	$ 10	$ 10

(money for all five years) and $10 million in *outlays* (money to be spent in the first year). The budget chart is shown in Figure 7. Congress acts on requests for budget authority, and grants that budget authority to the federal agencies which, in turn, spend the federal funds.

There are three main processes in each annual congressional budget cycle:

- Authorization
- Appropriations
- Budget Resolution.

The Authorization Process

In the authorization process, standing legislative committees of both chambers authorize the obligation of funds for specific programs. Authorizations specify the substance of federal programs, the agency that will implement them, and either the maximum dollar amount that may be spent to implement them, or the appropriation of "such sums as may be necessary" to run them. Authorizations generally have a definite time limit; renewal or modification of them is known as *re-authorization*. Some major programs are authorized (or re-authorized) annually, while others are authorized (or re-authorized) for several years at a time.

Authorizing responsibility for most health programs is divided among four congressional committees. In the House, authorizing jurisdiction relates to the source of funding. For example, the House Ways and Means Committee is responsible for programs funded from revenues raised through payroll taxes, such as Medicare and Social Security. On the other hand, the House Energy and Commerce Committee is primarily responsible for those health care programs funded through general revenues — e.g., block grants, Medicaid, and biomedical research.

In the Senate, the Finance Committee handles the Social Security Act, including Medicare, Medicaid, and maternal and child health programs. The Labor and Human Resources Committee authorizes spending for programs covered by the Public Health Service Act and other laws covering discretionary health programs.

The Nurse Education Act is authorized by the Energy and Commerce Committee in the House and the Labor and Human Resources Committee in the Senate. A more complicated example is the Stewart B. McKinney Homeless Assistance Act which, because of its numerous and diverse provisions, is authorized and re-authorized in the House by the Banking, Finance and Urban Affairs Committee; the Education and Labor Committee; the Energy and Commerce Committee; the Government Operations Committee; the Public Works and Transportation Committee; the Veterans' Affairs Committee, and the Ways and Means Committee. In the Senate, the authorizing committees are the Banking, Housing and Urban Affairs Committee; the Commerce, Science and Transportation Committee; the Finance Committee; the Governmental Affairs Committee; the Labor and Human Resources Committee, and the Veterans' Affairs Committee.

FIGURE 8   **FEDERAL APPROPRIATIONS SPENDING CAPS**
FY 1992 ($billions)

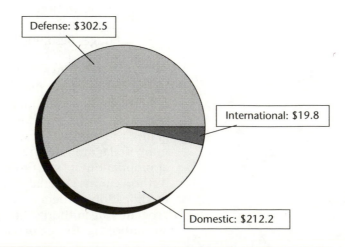

The Grassroots Lobbying Handbook

FIGURE 9

HEALTH CARE PROGRAM SPENDING FY 1992

FEDERAL APPROPRIATIONS ($billions)

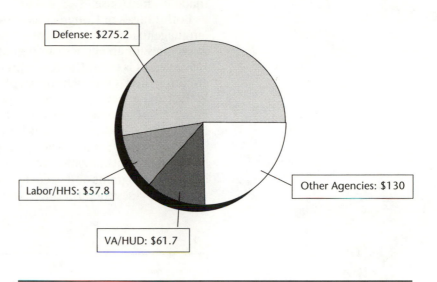

Defense: $275.2

Labor/HHS: $57.8

Other Agencies: $130

VA/HUD: $61.7

The Appropriations Process

The appropriations process determines how much funding each department, agency, or program is allocated for specific fiscal years. This can range from zero (which effectively kills the program for the fiscal year) up to the full authorization level.

Although the House and Senate appropriations committees are charged with the appropriations responsibility, in practice, much of the detailed work occurs on the subcommittee level (e.g., for both committees, the Labor, Health and Human Services subcommittees).

There are 13 appropriations subcommittees within both the House and Senate appropriations committees. Funds for most health programs are appropriated by the subcommittees on Labor, Health and Human Services. There are, however, several exceptions. For example, the Women, Infants, and Children (WIC) program is funded by the Agriculture appropriations subcommittees; Indian Health Services is funded by the Interior appropriations subcommittees; and veterans' health programs are funded by the Veterans' Affairs and housing and urban affairs and independent agencies appropriations subcommittees. The Medicaid program, which is an appropriated entitlement program, had a combined budget of federal and state funds of $158 billion in 1991 (See Figure 10).

The Constitution states that all revenue measures must originate in the House of Representatives, and, consequently, the House has the right to initiate all appropriations and taxation bills. In practical terms, this means that the House Appropriations Committee has the predominant role in crafting spending bills, while the Senate

Appropriations Committee serves as the "court of appeals" for agencies and interest groups that disagree with funding decisions made in the House.

Both houses of Congress have rules that bar attaching legislative language to appropriations measures (i.e., writing substantive policy guidelines for an agency or program into an appropriations bill). However, as is often the case with congressional rules, this one is circumvented. One such means of doing so is to *earmark* funds, within an agency's funding, for specific purposes; another is to attach *riders* to an appropriations bill, placing certain restrictions on funding (e.g. no Medicaid funds may be used for an abortion, except to save the life of the mother). These tactics blur the lines between the authorization process, which focuses on the operations of federal programs and agencies, and the appropriations process, which provides their funding.

FIGURE 10

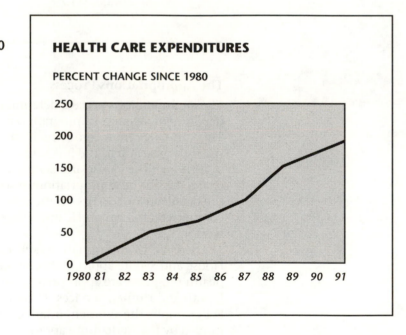

HEALTH CARE EXPENDITURES

PERCENT CHANGE SINCE 1980

Congress' concurrent budget resolution, passed each spring, limits the appropriations committees in the levels of funds they can appropriate. That resolution establishes targets for and ceilings on total federal spending and budget authority, and a floor on total revenues. The resolution also establishes targets for appropriations and other forms of spending for each of the twenty functional areas in the budget, of which "health" is one. The total and functional targets, when approved by Congress in the form of a concurrent resolution, provide guidance to the appropriations subcommittees and other spending committees on amounts available for the programs within their jurisdictions.

BUDGET PROCESS TIMETABLE

With the passage of the Budget Enforcement Act of 1990, the original 1974 budget process was amended and its timetable changed. The new calendar for congressional action on the budget appears below.

January	Congress convenes.
Five days before president's budget submission	CBO submits sequestration preview report for the fiscal year.
First Monday in February	President submits budget request to Congress, along with OMB sequestration preview report for the fiscal year.
Within 6 weeks after president's budget submission	All House and Senate standing committees submit "views and estimates" of expenditures for the coming year to their respective budget committees.
April 15	Statutory deadline for adoption of a budget resolution for the next fiscal year. (If a budget resolution has not been adopted by this date, the budget committees set spending limits for appropriations committees in discretionary categories that equal those set in the president's original budget submission.)
May 15	The House may start to debate and pass appropriations bills even if the budget resolution has not been adopted.
June 10	House Appropriations Committee must report out all appropriations bills by this date.
June 30	Congress completes action on all annual appropriations bills.
Prior to July 1	President must order a sequester within 15 days of enactment of appropriations that exceed a fiscal year's caps. If appropriations are enacted after July 1 that exceed the year's caps, the caps for the next fiscal year are lowered.
July 15	OMB submits mid-year budget review to Congress.
By August 10	The president must notify Congress if and how he or she plans to exempt military uniformed personnel from sequestration.
August 15	Congressional Budget Office submits its fiscal-year budget update.
August 20	OMB submits its sequestration update report.
October 1	All appropriations bills for the new fiscal year are to be enacted.
October 1	Fiscal year begins.
10 days after adjournment	Congressional Budget Office issues its final sequestration report.
15 days after adjournment	OMB issues its final sequestration report and the president issues any necessary sequestration order (which is effective immediately) to all federal departments and agencies.
30 days later	GAO sequester compliance report is due.

FIGURE 11

The budget committees review proposed levels of expenditures to determine if there will be a surplus or a deficit if all requests are approved and all taxes are collected. The budget committees also develop broad parameters for spending on program categories, which guide the appropriations committees as they determine specific program funding levels.

The Budget Resolution Process

In 1974, motivated by the impoundment of funds by President Richard M. Nixon and the desire to reassert its control over the budget process, Congress passed the Budget and Impoundment Control Act of 1974 (Public Law 93-344). Prior to the enactment of this legislation, total federal spending was the result of a chaotic series of uncoordinated authorization, appropriations, and revenue-raising measures. The Budget and Impoundment Control Act of 1974 made the following changes in the budget process:

- The fiscal year (FY) would begin on October 1 rather than July 1 to give Congress more time to study and discuss the budget.

- The House and Senate budget committees would be established to set economic priorities and make spending recommendations to the appropriations and revenue-raising (tax) committees, thereby injecting discipline into the budget process.

- The Congressional Budget Office (CBO) would be created to provide Congress with data and objective in-house advice on spending and taxes.

- Congress would have the right to review and approve presidential impoundment of funds.

- Congress would follow a timetable for passage of the budget.

At first, Congress adhered to the timetable outlined in the 1974 act. However, with the growing budget deficit of the 1980s, it began to ignore the timetable, and the government was funded more and more through *continuing resolutions* (a resolution passed by Congress and signed by the president that permits federal agencies to continue to operate — generally, at their current funding levels — until their regular appropriations bills are enacted). On several occasions, failure to enact either an appropriations bill or a continuing resolution has led to temporary shutdowns of the government.

To obtain better control over the growing deficit and to balance the federal budget, Congress passed the Balanced Budget and Emergency Deficit Control Act of 1985 (Public Law 99-177) (also known as the Gramm/Rudman/Hollings Act for the three senators who sponsored it). The major provisions of this act included:

- the goal of $0 in deficits by FY 1991;

- automatic cuts for non-exempt programs, to be divided equally between defense and non-defense targets if Congress failed to meet the deficit targets in a given fiscal year;

- exemptions from automatic cuts for certain programs (e.g., Social Security, Medicare, programs for the very poor such as Aid to

Families with Dependent Children and food stamps, and interest on the national debt); and,

- suspension of automatic cuts in time of war.

In 1987, Congress approved several changes to the Gramm/ Rudman/Hollings deficit reduction law including:

- extending the $0-deficit budget goal to FY 1993; and,
- stipulating that automatic spending cuts should be issued by the president with the recommendations of OMB.

In 1990, Congress and the administration sought to gain greater control over the budget, and the budget process was altered again when the Budget Enforcement Act of 1990 was enacted as Title XII of the Omnibus Budget Reconciliation Act of 1990 (Public Law 101-508). This law establishes a five-year procedure for deficit control, primarily by amending the Gramm/Rudman/Hollings Act and by adding new enforcement provisions to the Congressional Budget Act of 1974.

Title XII of Public Law 101-508 provided for several changes in the congressional budget process. The major shifts in that process are:

Five-year budgeting. Budget resolutions and necessary reconciliation bills will have to project spending revenues and deficits for five years.

Discretionary spending (yearly appropriated dollars) caps. Appropriations bills must stay below specific caps for defense, foreign, and domestic spending for fiscal years 1991-1993. For fiscal years 1994 and 1995, the law sets a single cap on all discretionary spending. Bills exceeding the caps will be considered out of order for floor consideration.(See Figure 12)

"Pay-as-you-go" entitlements and revenues. Any changes that Congress makes in taxes and mandatory spending (entitlement programs such as Medicare and food stamps) must be "deficit-neutral" (i.e., they cannot contribute to the deficit by reducing taxes or increasing spending without corresponding offsets). Tax cuts or entitlement increases must be paid for by tax increases or cuts in entitlement programs.

Exempted from the pay-as-you-go process. A number of programs were exempted from the pay-as-you-go process including:

- Social Security;
- Emergency direct spending (e.g., "Operation Desert Storm"); and,
- Increased spending for deposit insurance legislation (specifically, the savings-and-loan salvage operation).

Automatic cuts. If Congress exceeds the discretionary caps and violates the pay-as-you-go rule, OMB must order an across-the-board spending cut — or *sequester* — targeted at that part of the budget where the violation occurs. Such mini-sequesters also can be triggered by supplemental spending bills.

War and recession. A declaration of war would cancel sequestration. In addition, Congress could vote to cancel the sequestration process in the event of a projected recession or when economic growth is measured below one percent for two consecutive quarters.

Figure 12 contains the spending ceilings that apply in each of the categories during the first three years of the five-year plan. The limits for all discretionary programs will be combined for fiscal years 1994 and 1995.

FIGURE 12   **DISCRETIONARY SPENDING PROGRAM CAPS**

($ billions)

	FY 1991	FY 1992	FY 1993	FY 1994	FY 1995
Defense					
Budget Authority	288.90	301.72	291.48		
Outlays	297.70	308.18	296.96		
International					
Budget Authority	20.10	22.70	21.64		
Outlays	18.60	19.83	20.08		
Domestic					
Budget Authority	182.70	203.80	205.93		
Outlays	198.10	213.73	224.92		
Combined					
Budget Authority				510.09	524.98
Outlays				538.94	543.44

(Source: Congressional Budget Office)

Funding for all domestic discretionary programs will be permitted to grow by as much as inflation, unless an appropriations committee officially decides that an individual program should receive more or less than the inflation rate.

If a Member of Congress wants to create a new program or increase funding for an existing program by spending more money than is committed in the budget act's five-year plan, the amount of the new expenditure must be offset, either by proposing the creation of a new revenue source (e.g., new or increased taxes, or user fees) or by equal cuts in the spending for another program within the same budget authority category.

If congressional appropriations cause spending to exceed the discretionary spending caps or if legislation increases spending without an offsetting reduction, excess spending will be reduced by application of across-the-board cuts in each of the budget authority categories that are in violation of the law.

Non-discretionary (entitlement) programs. Under the changes enacted in Public Law 101-508, entitlement programs, such as

Medicare and Medicaid, must operate on a pay-as-you-go basis. Legislation enacting new spending must be offset by new revenues or reductions in another area of entitlement spending. Therefore, if Congress wants to expand Medicare benefits without raising additional revenues, offsetting reductions in other areas of the Medicare program would be needed.

Deficit targets. Public Law 101-508 also established new deficit targets for Fiscal Years 1991 through 1995 as follows:

FY 1991	$327 billion
FY 1992	$317 billion
FY 1993	$236 billion
FY 1994	$102 billion
FY 1995	$ 83 billion

THE FEDERAL REGULATORY PROCESS

After a bill becomes a law, it is sent to the federal agency responsible for writing the regulations to implement the law. Regulations have the force of law and are issued by agencies of the federal government under the authority delegated to them by a federal law or an executive order pursuant to law. Federal regulations are first printed in the *Federal Register*, and then codified annually by subject in the *Code of Federal Regulations (CFR)*.

FIGURE 13   **FEDERAL REGULATORY PROCESS**

- Congress passes law
- Agency writes implementing regulations
- Advanced notice of proposed rule making
- Proposed rule published
- Comment period
- Final rule issued
- Rule effective 30 days after final publication

Drafting of Regulations by Federal Agencies

The *Federal Register* informs the public about the activities of federal agencies. The Administrative Procedures Act (APA) requires that agencies publish regulations and general policy statements of organization and functions in the *Federal Register*. It contains agency regulations and legal notices, presidential proclamations and executive orders, and other administrative materials. It is published each federal working day.

The APA established a two-step procedure that an agency ordinarily uses for rule making. The rule making procedure applies only to substantive regulations. First, an agency must publish in the *Federal Register* a notice of proposed rule making, which contains:

1. The text of the proposed regulations or a description of the subjects and issues involved; and,

2. An invitation for the public to comment on the regulations.

After the proposed regulations have been published in the *Federal Register*, interested parties may submit written comments on them. Occasionally, the opportunity for comments may extend to testifying at a public hearing. A public hearing may be held on the agency's own initiative or because of a statutory requirement or a petitioner's request. Through written comments and/or testimony, concerned individuals and organizations bring to the agency's attention information on the proposed regulations that the agency may not have taken into account. The content of the final regulations may well be influenced by the views presented during this period.

The second step involves the careful consideration of the public's comments and, if the agency believes regulations are still necessary, the issuance of final regulations that take the comments into account.

Adoption and Release of Final Regulations

Final regulations are adopted only after the agency has reviewed the comments, made modifications, if any, to the draft regulations, and conducted further internal review. The final regulations, with a statement of their basis and purpose, are usually published in the *Federal Register* at least thirty days prior to their effective date, although exceptions to the time period are permitted under certain circumstances. If the final regulation does not concur with the comments received, a discussion of the rationale for the content of the final regulation is included. Occasionally, agencies may request additional public comment on a published final regulation. Regulations are subject to amendment or repeal petitions from concerned parties.

Final regulations are published periodically in the *CFR*, according to subject. Each subject is given a title number within the 50 titles of the *CFR*. Each title is revised annually.

Each revision of the *CFR* contains only regulations in force or those for which a future effective date has been established. If there have been intervening versions of any regulations since the previous edition, the *CFR* includes brief references to them, citing the issues and pages of the daily *Federal Register* in which they appeared. Regulations published in both the *Register* and *CFR* include citations of the statutory authority under which they were developed (also see pp. 17,19).

Notices

The day-to-day business of federal agencies is conducted by various means. The *Federal Register* may publish notices of hearings, investigations, advisory committee meetings, grant application information and deadlines, and other similar announcements. The monitoring of these notices in the *Federal Register* allows interested individuals, businesses, associations, and other organizations to compete for federal funds and express their views to the agency.

WHOM TO LOBBY: THE POWER PEOPLE

It is as important to know whom to lobby as to know where and when. Now that you are familiar with the processes in Congress and the federal agencies, it is time to look at the players.

You should know who your representatives and senators are, and have some information about them. As a constituent and a grass-roots lobbyist, you want to create your own personal biography of your representatives. You should know what committees they serve on and how powerful they are on those committees. This will tell you which legislation they may be able to influence. If possible, you should obtain a copy of their voting charts and a list of bills they have introduced and co-sponsored. These types of information can be obtained from your Member's office, the ANA Governmental Affairs Department, your SNA, and other associations to which you may belong. The Freedom of Information Act allows you to request information about which political action committees have contributed to the member's election or re-election and the amount of each contribution.

Know the strengths of your representatives. Are they respected by their colleagues? Are they well known or do they keep to themselves? How do other organizations rate them? Who are their friends — including colleagues in Congress as well as friends in their districts? Do they list a religion? If so, is this important to them? Each major religious denomination in the United States has a strong lobbying staff and membership and it is useful to know which Members will respond to these organizations.

It is always useful to know which causes a Member supports. There often are opportunities to assist with a Member's pet project — e.g., having a site in his or her district declared a historical landmark or a federal building named for an important local figure — and, in return, request support for one of your projects.

All Members maintain a Washington office as well as one or more district offices. Put in your file the addresses, telephone numbers, and facsimile machine (fax) numbers (if available) of each of those offices, so you may reach Members when they are in Washington and when they are home during recesses.

Finally, know the Member's staff. Most of the work of Congress is handled by the staff. Good relationships with them (both in Washington and in home states) give you invaluable contacts and a distinct advantage as a grassroots lobbyist.

LEADERSHIP IN THE CONGRESS

In both houses of Congress, there are several leadership positions. At the beginning of each Congress, the Members of each party in the House and Senate choose their leaders for the next two years.

In the House, every Democrat is a Member of the Democratic Caucus and every Republican belongs to the Republican Conference. The equivalent organizations in the Senate are the Republican and Democratic conferences. These groups elect the party leaders, approve committee assignments, and discuss party legislative strategies and policy.

The Constitution requires that there be a Speaker of the House of Representatives and a President and President Pro Tempore of the Senate. Over the years, other leadership positions have evolved in both chambers, specifically, the majority and minority leaders and the majority and minority whips. The Members of the leadership work for unity to achieve the legislative goals of their parties. Along with their leadership responsibilities come the benefits of large staffs, prime office space, higher salaries, priority in recognition during debate on the House and Senate floors, and greater media attention.

House of Representatives

Speaker of the House. The Speaker is the presiding officer of the House, and, as such, has tremendous influence over the scheduling of legislation and procedural maneuvers on the floor. This includes scheduling which bills are considered on the House floor, and when to remove a bill from the floor schedule because whip counts indicate that there are not sufficient votes to pass it.

The Speaker, second in the line of succession for the presidency after the vice president, is nominated by vote of the caucus of the majority party in the House (currently the Democratic Caucus). All 435 Members of the House must then vote on the majority party's nomination, but that vote is *pro forma* since the choice is strictly along party lines. A Democrat, as a Member of the majority party, has held the position of Speaker since 1955.

While the real power in the House was held by committee chairmen/chairwomen for most of the twentieth century, the position of Speaker has again become influential. In the mid-1970s, the Democratic Speaker became chairman/chairwoman of the party's Steering and Policy Committee, which assigns House Democrats to committees and nominates committee chairmen/chairwomen for vote by the caucus.

The Speaker also appoints all majority Members of the Rules Committee, which decides under what terms bills will be considered by the full House. In addition, the Speaker, in conjunction with the House parliamentarian, refers bills to committees. He or she may refer bills to more than one committee at a time, increasing the amount of time it takes for a bill to be acted upon, sometimes resulting in the death of legislation.

Majority Leader. At the beginning of each Congress, the majority leader is elected by secret ballot vote of the majority party caucus, currently the Democratic Caucus. The last five Speakers of the House served as majority leader for the Democrats before being elected Speaker, demonstrating one reason why this position is highly coveted.

The majority leader is the party's chief legislative strategist, promoting the party position on votes and working with the Speaker on the legislative schedule for the House.

Minority Leader. The leader of the minority party in the House is chosen by vote of the minority party, currently the Republican Conference. (The word, conference, in this case, as with the Democratic and Republican conferences in the Senate, is synonymous with caucus. It should not be confused with conference committees, part of the legislative process.)

The minority leader leads the opposition to the majority party's legislative program. When the president belongs to the same party, the minority leader also works closely with the administration to develop and promote administration-backed legislation. The minority leader, under these circumstances, also leads the fight to sustain presidential vetoes. If the president belongs to the same party as the congressional majority, the minority leader often is a major national spokesperson for the minority party.

Majority and Minority Whips. The term *whip* comes from foxhunting; the "whipper-in" is responsible for keeping the foxhounds from leaving the pack. Serving as an assistant to the majority or minority leader, the whip lobbies party Members for votes and works to obtain party unity on key legislative issues. Assisted by regional or zone whips, the whips make head counts for final votes, gather information regarding the party's overall attitude on an issue, and work to keep the party's membership in line. In 1991, the Democrats created three chief deputy-whips who are appointed by the Speaker of the House. The whip organizations are responsible for tracking weekly floor activity. The *Whip Notice,* published on Thursday or Friday of each week the House is in session, contains a list of the legislation to be considered on the House floor the following week.

The Democratic Whip is chosen by the Democratic Caucus and the Republican Whip is elected by the Republican Conference at the beginning of each Congress.

Senate

President of the Senate. The Constitution provides that the vice president serve as the president of the Senate. The president of the Senate rarely presides over that chamber and votes only to break a tie vote among the 100 senators. The position of president of the Senate is the only official participatory role that the executive branch has in Congress.

President Pro Tempore. The president pro tempore is charged by the Constitution with presiding over the Senate in the absence of the Senate president. He or she is elected by Members of the Senate and is traditionally the "dean" (i.e., most senior Member) of the majority party. Like the president of the Senate, the president pro tempore is a largely titular position, having very little power. However, the president pro tempore does participate in majority leadership meetings and is third in line for succession to the office of president of the United States (after the vice president and the Speaker of the House).

Majority Leader. Elected by the Senate Democratic or Republican conference (depending on which party is in the minority in the Senate at the beginning of each Congress), the Senate majority leader is responsible for scheduling bills on the floor and serves as chief strategist for passage of the party's legislative program.

Because Senate rules are fewer and less strict than those of the House, none of the presiding officers, including the majority leader, has the power that the Speaker of the House does to control debate.

Minority Leader. Elected by the Senate Democratic or Republican conference, the minority leader works for party unity to challenge the activities of the majority party. In the event that the president is a member of the same party, the minority leader guides the administration's legislative program through the Senate.

Party Whips. The positions and duties of majority and minority whip in the Senate are similar to those in the House. The whips work for party unity, count and predict votes on legislation, and assist their leaders in the scheduling of legislation for floor consideration and the lobbying of party colleagues. In the Senate, they also are responsible for ensuring that Members are present for cloture votes.

FIGURE 14　　**CONGRESSIONAL LEADERSHIP**

SENATE	HOUSE OF REPRESENTATIVES
• Vice President	• Speaker of the House
• President Pro Tempore	- Majority Leader
• Temporary presiding officer	- Majority Whip
	- 3 Chief Deputy Whips
• Majority Leader	
• Majority Whip	• Minority Leader
• Minority Leader	- Minority Whip
• Minority Whip	

CONGRESSIONAL STAFF

On Capitol Hill, one of the most significant changes in the last four decades has been the growth in the number and the influence of congressional staff. In 1930, approximately 1,400 people worked for representatives and senators as well as committees; in 1947, there were approximately 2,400 congressional staff. That number increased to 6,000 by 1960. Today, a work force of more than 20,000 includes Members' personal and committee staff, a police force, and a maintenance force, along with the staff who work for the congressional support agencies — the Congressional Research Service (CRS), a division of the Library of Congress; the Congressional Budget Office (CBO); the General Accounting Office (GAO); and the Office of Technology Assessment (OTA).

Given the complexity and diversity of legislative issues, it is almost impossible for any Member of Congress to be informed fully on every issue. Staff are usually the people to whom a senator or representative will turn first for assistance and advice. Congressional staff develop expertise on specific issues, the players and politics of the committees, the legislative process, and the interest groups and constituencies involved with legislation.

Congressional staff are a vital link between Members of Congress and constituents, lobbyists, and the public, as well as an essential element in the development and promotion of legislation. Remember: although staff members cannot vote, they have an indelible imprint on every other step in the legislative process. Members of Congress rely heavily on these employees and so should you. You should make every effort to work with, not circumvent, them.

A failure to develop a working relationship with congressional staff is detrimental to your cause for several reasons:

- Staff will be alienated because you did not trust them or feel they were important enough to work with.

- Staff will be blindsided when the Member asks them for advice and they are unprepared to respond because you have not kept them "in the loop."

- You will have lost an opportunity to obtain assistance and guidance from a valuable source.

- When the Member asks the staff for assistance and advice on your issue, the staff will not know to contact you or will be reluctant to contact you for further information if a relationship has not been established.

- While everyone values the opportunity to speak directly with senators and representatives on important issues, and to develop strong working relationships/friendships with them, congressional staff must be cultivated no less than the Members themselves. Because you are a constituent/lobbyist, the staff have a special obligation to answer your questions and respond to your requests. If you encounter a staff person who is uncooperative (the exception, not the rule), it is certainly your prerogative to go over that person's head to his or her supervisor. But do not discount all congressional staff members based on such an experience.

While there is no question that close ties to a Member — whether through personal friendship, campaign fund-raising, or being a constituent — are an essential component of any lobbying campaign, those ties can be greatly enhanced if a staff relationship also exists.

Personal Staff

There is a basic staff structure in all congressional offices, though it can vary among Members.

Administrative Assistant (AA). The AA acts as the executive assistant or chief of staff and often is in charge of overall office operations. He or she usually is the Member's political alter ego and is involved in all key political and policy decisions. The AA evaluates the political ramifications of legislative proposals and constituent requests and keeps the Member apprised of district and Capitol Hill political developments.

Legislative Assistant (LA). The LA focuses on particular policy issues, such as health, education, or taxes. Duties include keeping the Member abreast of developments in a specific legislative area; serving as liaison with the committee staff handling that topic (particularly if the Member is on that committee); handling constituent mail concerning the issue; meeting with constituents and lobbyists as the Member's personal representative on the issue of concern; and monitoring legislation and making recommendations to Members regarding the pros and cons of legislative proposals.

LAs often write the Member's speeches and position papers. In many offices, LAs are supervised by a *Legislative Director*, who is usually the senior legislative assistant. *Legislative Correspondents* handle the office's responses to routine constituent mail.

In Senate offices, where there are more staffers, a team of LAs in an office often will divide up and specialize in various issues, while in the House of Representatives, one or two LAs may handle all the legislation.

Caseworkers. Caseworkers resolve problems and answer inquiries from constituents regarding the federal government. A knowledge of federal agencies and departments is essential for this job, which includes finding lost Social Security checks, answering questions about federally financed student loans, and solving problems with veterans' retirement benefits. In recent years, many caseworkers have begun to work out of district — instead of Washington — offices where they can deal more directly and personally with constituents.

Press Secretary. The press secretary serves as the Member's chief spokesperson to the media. This staff member composes press releases dealing with legislative issues and other matters; writes newsletters; organizes press conferences, and decides the best medium through which to promote the Member's views on specific issues.

Executive/Personal Secretary. Because the executive/personal secretary schedules appointments and travel, he or she can be the most important person in gaining access to a senator or representative.

Office Manager. The office manager serves as the second-level manager in a congressional office and is in charge of handling clerical and computer system functions.

Receptionist. The receptionist serves as the first point of contact in a congressional office, answering the telephone, greeting visitors, arranging tours of the Capitol and White House for constituents, and providing Washington, DC tourist information.

District Office Staff

Every Member has at least one office in his or her home district or state, and it usually is located in a federal building. These offices work directly with constituents on a daily basis and should be contacted if you wish to invite a senator or representative to speak at or participate in a local event. A personal tour of a local hospital or medical center, school, or factory can be of tremendous value in promoting desired legislation. If the Member cannot accept an invitation, a staff member from the district office may attend on his or her behalf.

Committee Staff

Most committees and subcommittees have both a majority and minority staff. They advise Members during hearings and mark-up sessions and assist in the floor debate during final consideration of a bill. Committee staff members for the majority play a larger role than their minority party counterparts in setting legislative agendas. Promoting legislation and gaining access to the committee Members is possible through contact with the committee or subcommittee staff.

The basic committee and subcommittee staff structures are as discussed below.

The staff director and general counsel. The staff director and general counsel are closely allied with the committee or subcommittee chairman/chairwoman. They work closely with Members and staff of both chambers, interest groups, and agency officials to facilitate or obstruct the passage of legislation.

Professional staff. The professional staff serve as policy specialists and analysts in a particular legislative/issue area and provide the necessary legislative expertise to Members of the committee.

Press secretary. The press secretary promotes media coverage of the committee's activities.

FIGURE 15   **CONGRESSIONAL STAFF**

PERSONAL STAFF	COMMITTEE STAFF
Administrative Assistant	Staff Director
Legislative Director	Counsel
Legislative Assistants	Professional Staff/
Legislative Correspondents	Policy Analysts
Press Secretary	Press Secretary
Case Workers	Administrative
Personal Secretary/	
Executive Secretary	
Office Manager	
Receptionist	

Administrative staff. The administrative staff arrange the hearing rooms, organize the office and committee publications, and oversee the committee's budget and expenses.

LEGISLATIVE SUPPORT AGENCIES

The staff members of the CRS, the CBO, the GAO, and the OTA are additional sources of information for senators and representatives and personal and committee staff. They provide expertise in myriad areas — from MX missiles to alternative energy sources, from the savings and loan crisis to health care reform. Unlike the personal and committee staffs, they are nonpartisan and are hired to give objective advice and information to any Member who makes a request.

GOVERNMENT PRINTING OFFICE

The GPO was established in 1861 to act as a public printer for the federal government (including Congress). Most federal publications are available from the GPO by mail. Individuals and organizations may establish an account to purchase publications. Information regarding orders may be obtained from:

> **Superintendent of Documents**
> **Government Printing Office**
> **Washington, DC 20402**
> **(202) 783-3238**

CONGRESSIONAL COMMITTEES: THE HEART OF CONGRESS

" . . . it is not far from the truth to say that Congress in session is Congress on public exhibition, while Congress in its committee rooms is Congress at work."

— Woodrow Wilson

Committees are the heart of the legislative process. Their deliberations are where the nuts-and-bolts legislative work is done. Committees have existed in the House and Senate since 1789, allowing for an orderly division of work and consideration of legislation. The size of the House and Senate, coupled with the large number of bills introduced each year (about 5,000), makes it impossible for Members of Congress to assess all pieces of legislation adequately. Consequently, it falls to committees to analyze the legislation within their jurisdictions. In turn, most committees have established subcommittees to allow for a further division of work.

Committees have enormous power. They hold hearings, conduct investigations, oversee government programs, write and initiate bills, approve bills, report bills to the floor, and kill legislation, either through inaction or defeat. The vast majority of legislation enacted into law first received subcommittee and committee approval.

There are three basic types of committees: *standing committees*, which are permanent and have broad legislative mandates; *select* or *special committees*, which are temporary and established to address a specific issue area for a certain period of time (these committees have an investigative role and usually no legislative authority); and *joint committees* — comprised of a specified number of both House and Senate Members — which study and report on specific policy issues.

The fact that there are nearly eight times as many committees and subcommittees in Congress today (approximately 300) as there were in 1947 (38), often causes legislative "gridlock." On August 1, 1991, the *Washington Post* reported that, on one Wednesday during the previous month, the newspaper,

"needed 26 reporters just to visit 57 committee and subcommittee hearings, excluding appropriations. The hearings dealt with everything from the annual oversight of the Internal Revenue Service to a proposed third airport for metropolitan Chicago. Reporters interviewed one Member who showed up at the wrong hearing because too many appointments 'had twisted his schedule into knots'." ("Reforming Congress by Committee," Guy Gugliotta [*Washington Post,* August 1, 1991, A13]).

Majority- and minority-party membership ratios on committees are determined at the beginning of each Congress. Generally, they are based on the ratios of Democrats to Republicans in each chamber. Members are assigned to committees by caucuses/conferences of the respective parties and these assignments are confirmed by a vote of the full chamber. The majority Member having the most years of service on the committee usually is designated as *chairman/chairwoman*, and the minority party Member with the most years is usually the *ranking minority Member*. Subcommittee positions are determined in the same manner, with the full committee determining subcommittee Membership and maintaining the same majority/minority ratios.

The majority staff of a committee are hired by the chairman/chairwoman; the minority staff are hired by the ranking minority Member.

The chairman/chairwoman usually has earned his or her position by long service on a particular committee and has developed an expertise on the issues that come before the committee. Although the chairman/chairwoman traditionally is the most senior Member of the committee, following congressional reforms of the 1970s, this is no longer an ironclad rule. Chairmen/Chairwomen must now stand for election by their party caucus/conference and, on several occasions, the most senior Member of the majority party has been passed over in favor of another Member whose views may be more in line with a majority of Members of his or her party, or who is deemed to be more physically capable of handling the grueling job of committee chairman/chairwoman.

The days of the autocratic committee chairmen, who could run their committees as they wished, are over. Committee heads must now answer to their fellow party Members. These changes have resulted in a more democratic committee process, in which the chairman/chairwoman will negotiate scheduling of legislation and other important matters with both the ranking minority Member and other Members of the committee.

Committee chairmen/chairwomen have wide discretion in establishing the legislative priorities of committees. They control the agenda, refer legislation to subcommittees, manage committee funds, and control committee staff. Chairmen/Chairwomen are deciding voices in determining whether a proposal will receive consideration by their committees. A bill can languish in committee if the chairman/chairwoman is opposed to the proposal. For example, a bill mandating a study of the federal wage system, looking for sex- and race-based wage discrimination, was bottlenecked because the chairman of the Senate Governmental Affairs Committee opposed the concept of pay equity. It was not until there was a change in the majority party in the Senate and, correspondingly, a new chairman of the committee, that hearings were held, and the bill reported to the full Senate.

House Members usually serve on two committees. However, if a Member serves on the Appropriations, Rules, or Ways and Means committee, that usually is his or her only standing committee assignment. Generally, senators serve on two "A" (major legislative) committees and one "B" (lower-ranking) committee.

Traditionally, the most sought after committees in the House have been Appropriations, Rules, and Ways and Means. The popularity of some committees ebbs and flows; however, Appropriations, and Ways and Means always have been highly prized because they have jurisdiction over money and revenue matters. In the 1980s, these taxing and spending committees were thrust even farther into the limelight because of Congress' growing tendency to pile most of its legislative work on to just a few fiscal measures, thereby ensuring congressional passage and presidential signature. In the last decade, the Budget, and Energy and Commerce committees also have become popular.

In the Senate, the most popular committees traditionally have been Appropriations and Finance, while the Budget and Armed Services committees also have been in demand recently. Members of the House and Senate Budget committees can serve on those committees for only six years and, hence, membership is rotated on a prescribed schedule.

Once a bill has been referred to committee, the committee can hold hearings, debate, *mark up* (amend), and *report* (approve) a bill, sending it to the full House or Senate for consideration. A committee also can rewrite a bill in its entirety, combine two or more bills into one proposal, refuse to even consider a bill, or consider and reject a bill. If a committee fails to act on a bill prior to the adjournment of a Congress, the bill dies.

When a committee does report out a bill, the basic structure of that bill usually is maintained through the rest of the legislative process. This is because committee Members and their staffs have substantial expertise on the subjects under the committee's jurisdiction and other Members respect their judgement on specific legislative proposals. Numerous floor amendments to a carefully crafted committee bill tend to be rare, especially in the House.

A committees's decision not to report a bill usually is respected by the chamber as a whole, though, in recent years, one exception to this rule has been the case of judicial nominations. Only the Senate Judiciary Committee considers federal court nominations, including those to the Supreme Court. (The House of Representatives has no constitutional authority to consider presidential nominations.)

In 1987, the Senate Judiciary Committee failed to approve the nomination of Judge Robert Bork to the Supreme Court. Since the administration did not withdraw the nomination, it proceeded to the full Senate for consideration, where it was defeated. In 1991, the Senate Judiciary Committee reported the Supreme Court nomination of Judge Clarence Thomas to the full Senate with no recommendation (because the committee had split its vote — 7 for and 7 against — on the nomination). Despite this action, the Senate approved the nomination by a vote of 52 yeas to 48 nays.

Notwithstanding the reforms of recent years, however, committee chairmen/chairwomen still wield great power on Capitol Hill. An example of this clout was the 1986 tax reform bill. When the House Ways and Means Committee mark-up of that bill bogged

down in 1985, Chairman Dan Rostenkowski (D-IL) broke the
deadlock with tough back-room negotiations among the Democrats
on the committee.

During Senate Finance Committee consideration of tax reform
in 1986, that committee's chairman, Bob Packwood (R-OR), sus-
pended mark-up of the bill when it became apparent that he was
going to lose votes in the committee on several of his key proposals. Packwood and the staff director of the committee then met
privately in a Capitol Hill restaurant, came up with a new tax
strategy, and met with a core group of senators to craft a bill to take
back to the full committee. House/Senate conference agreement
was reached only after a series of lengthy, closed-door negotiations
between chairmen Rostenkowski and Packwood.

THE HEARING PROCESS

An important part of the committee process is the *hearing*. A
hearing is a fact-finding mission to obtain information and solicit
opinions on pending legislation from officials of the executive
branch, other Members of Congress, representatives of interest
groups, academic experts, and individual citizens. Hearings are a
major step toward the enactment of legislation. The decision to
hold a hearing on a legislative proposal often symbolizes its importance. It is rare (except for technical and minor bills) that legislation
proceeds to the Senate or House floor without first being the subject
of scrutiny in one or more hearings.

Since committee chairmen/chairwomen and their staffs have the
ability to select the subject matter and invite the witnesses, the tone
of a hearing may determine the direction of future debate on a
legislative proposal. All spoken and written statements become a
part of the permanent public hearing record.

If you are a constituent of a Member who serves on a committee
scheduling a particular hearing, you can request to testify. You
must be aware, however, that travel to Washington, DC to present
the oral testimony usually is at your own expense. It also is your
responsibility to comply with committee requirements to submit at
least 50 copies of your testimony (sometimes 100, or even 200) to
the committee staff at least 48 hours in advance of the hearing.

If the subject is a popular or controversial one, it is likely that
more people than time allows will request to testify . In these cases,
the committee chairman/chairwoman will determine which witnesses will be allowed to deliver oral testimony. For example,
hearings on health care reform currently are very popular, and
testimony by provider groups often has been limited to three
organizations: the ANA, the American Medical Association (AMA),
and the American Hospital Association (AHA). As hearings on this
subject continue, other provider groups will be able to present oral
testimony.

Despite limits on the number of witnesses actually presenting
testimony, committees will always accept all written testimony. As
a concerned citizen or member of a SNA, it is your right to submit a

written statement to be included in the official record. That way, your opinion will be read by committee Members, committee staff, and other individuals who examine the written record. It is a relatively easy way to lobby congressional committees on a particular bill or issue.

Check with committee staff prior to submitting your statement to ascertain the appropriate format, the number of copies required (generally five to ten), and the correct address to which to send them. Many committees have a rule that any statement not in compliance with their guidelines will not be printed in the hearing record, but will be maintained in the committee files for review and use by the committee.

Committee chairmen/chairwomen may occasionally decide to take congressional hearings "on the road," holding them somewhere other than Washington, DC (*field hearings*). These often are held in the home district or state of either the committee chairman/chairwoman or another committee Member. If a congressional hearing of interest is held in your state, it is an effective lobbying strategy to request to testify.

The format for hearings is fairly uniform for all committees. Witnesses usually appear on a panel with two or three other individuals. Most oral statements are limited to five minutes per witness. After the entire panel has finished delivering oral testimony, each committee Member has the opportunity to question each witness. Except for controversial witnesses or administration representatives, most witnesses do not face extensive questioning.

Recently, more and more celebrities have testified, drawing attention to certain issues that otherwise might not be newsworthy. More people and press attended a recent hearing on family farms and the problems facing small farmers — featuring testimony from Jessica Lange, Sissy Spacek, and Jane Fonda (they had all appeared in recent movies about life on a farm) — than almost any other hearing in congressional history.

Hearings can be used to demonstrate support for a particular legislative proposal. This is why committees solicit witnesses who may represent a broad-based coalition. For example, if you can indicate that you not only represent a SNA, but, also, a specialty nursing association in your state, and/or other health and consumer interest groups, the influence of your statement will increase.

Committee Members always look for support for their individual bills. It is important to remember that the committee often will want to solicit your expert opinion as a health care practitioner, but will also want your organization's official endorsement of a legislative proposal. It is not necessary to endorse a proposal in order to present or submit testimony, but it is useful to be aware of committee Members' bills on the subject prior to presenting your oral testimony. You may be asked by a Member about his or her bill. Be prepared!

There are many other types of committees to whom it is useful to present testimony. For example, all state legislatures have some form of committee process, and it is equally important to be known in your state as a health care expert and to be available to testify on these matters before your state legislature's committees. Many states have other types of committees (such as commissions on women, state health advisory boards, and safety committees) which hold hearings. Although action by such committees does not have the force of state or federal law, these groups are useful forums for presenting your organization's positions on specific issues. These hearings are often covered by local media or followed by official reports which are subsequently submitted to the state legislature for review.

HEALTH-RELATED COMMITTEES

There are nine standing committees in the Congress with primary jurisdiction over health-related legislation. They are the Senate Appropriations, Budget, Finance, and Labor and Human Resources committees; and the House Appropriations, Budget, Education and Labor, Energy and Commerce, and Ways and Means committees. In addition, the Veterans' Affairs committees of both chambers have jurisdiction over the veterans' health care system. (There also are select committees which examine health-related matters — e.g., the select committees on aging — but these committees have no authority to act on legislation.)

Because of the scope and importance of health-related legislation, many other committees may have jurisdiction over portions of health bills. They would consider those sections of the legislation which fall within their purview.

If your senators and representatives serve on these committees, they are well-placed to influence health policy. Although committee membership changes in each Congress, most Members remain on powerful committees and, when a vacancy does occur, there generally is a great deal of maneuvering to fill it.

The relative importance of individual committees vis-a-vis health issues and legislation varies with circumstances. Alterations in committee jurisdictions, the personality and legislative interests of the committee chairmen/chairwomen and the individual committee Members, as well as the public's interest in a particular health issue — all pay a role in determining which committees are most likely to have the greatest impact on a particular health issue or proposal in a given year.

The jurisdictions and responsibilities of the nine major health committees and their relevant subcommittees — as well as those other committees which handle health-related issues — are described below.

- **Health-Related Committees in the Senate**

  Committee on Appropriations
  S-128, The Capitol
  Washington, DC 20510
  (202) 224-3471

  Jurisdiction: Appropriation of funds for executive agencies and federal programs and activities.

Appropriations Subcommittee on Labor, Health and Human Services, Education, and Related Agencies
SD-186 Dirksen Senate Office Building
Washington, DC 20510
(202) 224-7283

Jurisdiction: Department of Education (except Native American education); Department of Health and Human Services (except Food and Drug Administration, Indian Health Service, and Office of Consumer Affairs); Department of Labor; ACTION (domestic programs); Corporation for Public Broadcasting; Federal Mine Safety and Health Review Commission; National Commission on Libraries and Information Science; National Council on the Handicapped; National Labor Relations Board; Occupational Safety and Health Review Commission; Physician Payment Review Commission; Propsective Payment Assessment Commission; and the Railroad Retirement Board.

Committee on the Budget
SD-621 Dirksen Senate Office Building
Washington, DC 20510
(202) 224-0642

Jurisdiction: Coordination of spending and revenues in the federal budget; to make continuing studies of the effect on budget outlays of relevant existing and proposed legislation and to report the results of such studies to the Senate on a regular basis; to request and evaluate continuing studies of tax expenditures; to review the conduct of the Congressional Budget Office; to consider impoundment legislation; and to consider matters affecting the congressional budget process.

Committee on Finance
SD-205 Dirksen Senate Office Building
Washington, DC 20510
(202) 224-4515

Jurisdiction: Taxes, tariffs, trade, Old-Age and Survivors Insurance (Social Security), Medicare, Medicaid, unemployment insurance, and general revenue sharing.

Committee on Labor and Human Resources
SD-428 Dirksen Senate Office Building
Washington, DC 20510
(202) 224-5375

Jurisdiction: Education, labor, health, and public welfare; labor standards and labor statistics; wages and hours of labor; child labor; regulation of foreign laborers; handicapped individuals; equal employment opportunity; occupational safety and health; private pensions; aging; public health; biomedical research and development; student loans; and domestic activities of the American Red Cross.

Committee on Veterans' Affairs
SR-414 Russell Senate Office Building
Washington, DC 20510
(202) 224-9126

Jurisdiction: Veterans' measures including pensions; life insurance; compensation of veterans; vocational rehabilitation and education; veterans' hospitals, medical care, and national cemeteries.

Select Committee on Indian Affairs
SH-838 Hart Senate Office Building
Washington, DC 20510
(202) 224-2251

Jurisdiction: Conducting studies of any and all matters pertaining to problems and opportunities of Native Americans, including Native-American land management and trust responsibilities and Native American education, health, special services, and loan programs.

Special Committee on Aging
SD-G31 Dirksen Senate Office Building
Washington, DC 20510
(202) 224-5364

Jurisdiction: Conducting studies of any and all matters pertaining to problems and opportunities of older people, including problems and opportunities of maintaining health, assuring adequate income, finding employment, engaging in productive and rewarding activity, securing proper housing, and, when necessary, obtaining care or assistance.

- **Health-Related Committees in the House of Representatives**

  Committee on Appropriations
  H-218 Capitol
  Washington, DC 20515
  (202) 225-2771

  Jurisdiction: Appropriation of funds for executive agencies and federal programs and activities.

  > **Appropriations Subcommittee on Labor, Health and Human Services, Education, and Related Agencies**
  > 2358 Rayburn House Office Building
  > Washington, DC 20515
  > (202) 225-3508
  >
  > *Jurisdiction*: Department of Education (except Native American education); Department of Health and Human Services (except Food and Drug Administration, Indian Health Service, and Office of Consumer Affairs); Department of Labor; ACTION; Corporation for Public Broadcasting; Federal Mine Safety and Health Review Commission; National Commission on Libraries and Information Science; National Council on Disability; National Labor Relations Board; Occupational Safety and Health Review Commission; Propsective Payment Assessment Commission; Physician Payment Review Commission; Soldiers' and Airmen's

Home; U.S. Naval Home; United States Institute of Peace; Federal Mediation Service; National Commission on AIDS; Railroad Retirement Board; National Mediation Board.

Committee on the Budget
214 O'Neill House Office Building (Annex I)
Washington, DC 20515
(202) 226-7200

Jurisdiction: Coordination of spending and revenues in the federal budget.

Committee on Education and Labor
2181 Rayburn House Office Building
Washington, DC 20515
(202) 225-4527

Jurisdiction: education; labor; child labor; labor standards; labor statistics; mediation and arbitration of labor disputes; food programs for children in schools; vocational rehabilitation; wages and hours of labor; welfare of minors.

Committee on Energy and Commerce
2125 Rayburn House Office Building
Washington, DC 20515
(202) 225-2927

Jurisdiction: Foreign and interstate commerce; national energy policy; energy resources, information and technology; Department of Energy; railroads; inland waterways; interstate and foreign communications; travel and tourism; securities and exchange; consumer affairs and protection; Medicaid; health care and health facilities (except health care supported by payroll deductions [i.e., Medicare]); biomedical research and development.

Energy and Commerce Subcommittee on Health and the Environment
2415 Rayburn House Office Building
Washington, DC 20515
(202) 225-4952

Jurisdiction: Public health and quarantine; hospital construction; mental health and research; biomedical programs and health protection in general, including Medicaid and national health insurance; foods and drugs; drug abuse; Clean Air Act; environmental protection.

Committee on Veterans' Affairs
335 Cannon House Office Building
Washington, DC 20515
(202) 225-3527

Jurisdiction: Veterans' measures including cemeteries; compensation; life insurance; pensions; compensation; and veterans' hospitals and medical care.

Committee on Ways and Means
1102 Longworth House Office Building
Washington, DC 20515
(202) 225-3625

Jurisdiction: Taxation; Social Security; tariffs; trade; health care programs financed through payroll taxes (Medicare); tax-exempt foundations; and revenue measures.

Ways and Means Subcommittee on Health
1114 Longworth House Office Building
Washington, DC 20515
(202) 225-7785

Jurisdiction: Bills and matters relating to programs which provide payments for health care, health delivery systems, or health research; bills and matters relating to the Medicare program; tax credit and deduction provisions of the Internal Revenue Code relating to health insurance premiums and health care costs.

Select Committee on Aging
712 O'Neill House Office Building (Annex I)
Washington, DC 20515
(202) 226-3375

Jurisdiction: Problems of older Americans including income mainte-nance, housing, health, welfare, employment, education, recre-ation, and participation in family and community life.

Select Committee on Children, Youth, and Families
385 Ford House Office Building (Annex II)
Washington, DC 20515
(202) 226-7660

Jurisdiction: Conducting a continuing and comprehensive study and review of problems of children, youth, and families including, but not limited to income maintenance, health (including medical and child development research), nutrition, education, welfare, employ-ment and recreation.

LOBBYING STRATEGIES AND GRASSROOTS TECHNIQUES

At this point, you should be familiar with your issues, the legisla-tive and regulatory processes, and the people you will be lobbying. This section addresses the heart of this book — the techniques to use in your lobbying campaign. No one technique, plan, or strategy is better than another; your lobbying plan should include several different types of action, taking place, preferably, at different stages of the legislative and regulatory processes (See **A Step-by-Step Grassroots Lobbying Strategy Guide** p. 72).

The key is to have a plan. Outline on a work sheet the actions you propose and an approximate time frame for accomplishing them, providing yourself with a working plan, as well as a chronological record of your accomplishments. You also will want to record the reactions and responses you receive from elected and appointed officials.

FIGURE 16

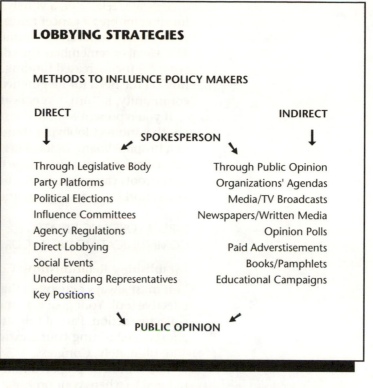

LOBBYING STRATEGIES

METHODS TO INFLUENCE POLICY MAKERS

DIRECT   **INDIRECT**

SPOKESPERSON

DIRECT	INDIRECT
Through Legislative Body	Through Public Opinion
Party Platforms	Organizations' Agendas
Political Elections	Media/TV Broadcasts
Influence Committees	Newspapers/Written Media
Agency Regulations	Opinion Polls
Direct Lobbying	Paid Adverstisements
Social Events	Books/Pamphlets
Understanding Representatives	Educational Campaigns
Key Positions	

PUBLIC OPINION

If you contact your Member and he or she is receptive to your proposal, there is no need to lobby that Member again until the crucial vote is scheduled. At that point, you will want to contact him or her with a reminder of your continued interest and thanks for his or her position. Other Members may need more intense lobbying efforts.

Now, you are ready to lobby. There are two basic types of lobbying — *direct* and *indirect* (see Figure 16).

INDIRECT LOBBYING STRATEGIES

Indirect lobbying strategies can be very effective. As a grassroots lobbyist, you can indirectly lobby by influencing public opinion, which, in turn, will influence policy makers. Public opinion plays a very large role in persuading policy makers; after all, they are supposed to represent their constituents.

An example of an indirect lobbying effort would be launching an education or media campaign on breast cancer awareness by persuading local radio stations to broadcast public service messages on mammography screening. Then, a local newspaper might pick up on the radio spots and write an editorial on the need for Medicaid funding for mammographies for low-income women. Every congressional office subscribes to every paper published in its district, as well as the major papers published in the state. A legislative assistant may read the editorial and bring it to the attention of his or her Member. In addition, the editorial may prompt some constituents to write to their representatives.

Several weeks later, a vote is held in the House on increasing funding for breast cancer research and raising the income cap for poor women to receive mammography screening under Medicaid. The Member remembers the editorial, along with the letters, and votes for the increased funding. You have educated your community on the need for heightened awareness of breast cancer, and the community, in turn, has educated the Member.

If you represent a small constituency or have limited resources, another indirect lobbying strategy is to lobby a larger organization, or a hospital board, or local health association to take a stand on a particular issue and encourage them to use their resources to mount a grassroots campaign. With this strategy, one person spearheads a large effort by encouraging others to adopt the same agenda.

DIRECT LOBBYING STRATEGIES: COMMUNICATING WITH YOUR LEGISLATOR

Establishing Relationships: Constituents Count

You must always remember that constituent pressure is a very effective tool. Your goal is to mobilize a group of individuals for collective action. Part of this strategy must involve educational efforts — educating your grassroots lobby corps, the general public, and, ultimately, Congress.

You should be prepared to use different lobbying strategies tailored to where your proposal is in the legislative and regulatory process. No one strategy should be implemented throughout a lobbying campaign. The rules on lobbying federal agencies and the judiciary differ from those concerning Congress. Though it is your responsibility as a grassroots lobbyist to express your opinions on matters of public policy, it is illegal to lobby federal judges and you must be careful in your approaches to government officials.

When a bill is pending in Congress or a state legislature, you will want to write letters. If your bill has been enacted into law and is waiting for regulations to be drafted by a federal or state agency, you will want to comment on the proposed regulations. There is no use in getting a bill through Congress, if the final regulations do not reflect congressional intent. You must see the process through from beginning to end. If the law has been challenged in court and is being considered by the Supreme Court, you may want to file an *amicus curiae* (literally, "friend of the court") brief to explain why you believe your interpretation of the law is correct.

Even within one step of the process, you may need to implement different strategies. For example, your lobbying techniques could differ depending upon whether a bill is being considered in committee or being debated by the full House or Senate.

The first step in a successful direct lobbying campaign is to communicate effectively with legislators.

Communicating with Your Legislator: The General Rules

Although Congress' day-to-day activities may seem chaotic, there is a definite order and set of rules governing the proceedings. Utilizing these rules, you can be a very effective lobbyist.

Congress tends to be a reactive institution. It reacts to crisis — whether real or perceived — including constituent pressure. As a lobbyist, you can create this pressure with a public education campaign. By involving the public, you create the pressure needed to force Congress to act. An example of such pressure occurred with the Medicare Catastrophic Act. Congress passed a bill one year, but as a result of a group of elderly voters protesting loudly, repealed the law, through new legislation, eighteen months later.

As an institution, the Senate is more insulated and less reactive than the House. This can be attributed partly to the fact that senators are elected only every six years whereas House Members are elected every two. This election cycle makes the Senate less anxious about reacting immediately. In addition, because of the differences in House and Senate rules governing floor debate (House floor proceedings are more regulated and debate time is always limited), the Senate takes a longer time to consider an issue.

Members tend to hear from people who are dissatisfied, rather than satisfied, with the status quo. Consequently, Members may be led to believe, incorrectly, that large numbers of their constituents disagree with an issue. It is very important to tell a Member when you are happy with an action he or she took, as well as when you are unhappy.

There will always be "sacred cows" in Congress — issues that Members tiptoe around. For example, issues that have an impact on the elderly, such as Social Security and Medicare, are dealt with very cautiously. This is, in large part, because the elderly population is large and an influential lobbying group. Generally, the elderly are informed and often have time to contact their Members. As the population ages, the political power of senior citizens will become even stronger.

Remember, you must have a strategy to influence every step of the congressional and regulatory process. Because of the defensive nature of Congress, advancing legislation is more complicated than blocking it. To go from the draft of a bill, to congressional consideration, to signature by the president can take many years.

It may take a very long time just for Congress to pass a bill. To adopt a new child care program took four years; to gain reimbursement for nurse practitioners under the federal employees' health-benefits systems took five years; a proposal for a family and medical leave policy took over eight years, and health care reform may take a decade. *Persistence and patience are the two key factors in lobbying.*

Always be ready to compromise; it is the key element in the enactment of most legislation. First drafts of legislation rarely represent the final law. For example, the first version of the eventual Family and Medical Leave Act passed in Congress would have provided twenty-six weeks of leave for parents of newborn, newly adopted, or seriously ill children (for employers with five or more employees). The final version of the same legislation, signed into law by the president in February 1993, provides twelve weeks of leave (for employers with fifty or more employees).

Using the Congressional Calendar.

Whether you are arranging a personal visit or a phone call, you should know when your Member is in a recess or *district work period*. For Members to spend time in their districts with their constituents, the House and Senate both have long recesses around holidays. Because the purpose of these district work periods is for the Member to meet with his or her constituents, they are when you should schedule your appointments. In addition, most Members return to their home states on Friday afternoons and return to Washington on Monday afternoons. For this reason, few floor votes are scheduled on Mondays or Fridays.

Congress traditionally convenes in early January each year, although Members often shuttle back to their home districts throughout January. Ten-day recesses usually are scheduled around Presidents' Day, Easter, Memorial Day, and the Fourth of July. Congress normally goes home in early August and reconvenes after Labor Day. Four- or five-day breaks are taken for Rosh Hashanah, for Yom Kippur, and for Columbus Day. In election years, Congress adjourns in early- to mid-October. (Congress reconvening after the election is known as a *lame duck session*). In non-election years, Congress tries to adjourn prior to Thanksgiving, although the session rarely ends before mid-December.

If an issue is scheduled for debate and a vote after a recess, the most effective lobbying strategy would have the grassroots lobbyists meeting with the Member in the home district during that recess, and the organization's Washington lobbyist following up with a visit to the Member when Congress reconvenes. During this time, letters also are helpful.

The Congressional Calendar is printed in early January and is available from your representative's and/or senators' offices. The House and Senate recess schedules generally vary only slightly.

In any communication with your legislator, there are several points to remember:

Do Your Homework.

Be sure you have reviewed the material and information you want to discuss. Whether your supporting evidence consists of personal illustrations or hard data, verify its accuracy.

Learn as much as possible about your legislator's views on the issue you plan to discuss. For example, if your legislator does not support a change in the Nurse Practice Act, find out why. What are his or her concerns, and how has he or she reacted to previous requests for support? Is the legislator opposed to the general concept behind a certain legislative proposal (e.g., mandated benefits) or does the legislator just oppose a technical component (e.g., a review board)? Is there room for a compromise?

Review your strategies for effectiveness.

Identify Yourself.

When you present yourself to your legislator, identify yourself as:

1. *A constituent.* Include the name of the city, county, congressional district, or state where you reside.

2. *A health care professional.* Include any relevant information that may be useful (e.g., "I am a nurse practitioner in private practice and, therefore, I am knowledgeable about small businesses."). This type of information lends credibility to your views and/or request.

3. *A member of a large group, organization, or coalition* (e.g., "I am a member of the Iowa Nurses Association."). This information suggests strength in numbers. The legislator will assume you are in contact with other members of your group (i.e., voters).

Be Specific.

If you know the number of a bill or public law, use it. Because it is not unusual for several versions of the same proposal to be introduced, it is helpful to refer to a specific bill number. For example, in the 102nd Congress, over 50 bills that addressed health care reform were introduced. If you are interested in a specific proposal, cite it. Be specific about the type of action you are requesting. Do you want the Member to co-sponsor the bill, hold hearings on a legislative proposal, or vote in a specific manner?

Look for the Member to make a commitment. Ask for the Member's position on an issue. Don't let him or her "slip, slide, and duck" around it. You will note that many legislators will discuss a bill in a reply letter without ever indicating their position. Phrases such as, "I am studying the issue" or, "I will keep your views in mind" are common. If a Member of Congress or other legislator indicates his or her support for an issue, hold him or her to that promise.

Be Concise.

Time is of the essence for both the legislator and his or her staff. Keep letters to one page. If you are enclosing supporting documentation, try to trim it down to a one- or two-page fact sheet. Huge notebooks wind up in the trash can. A concise fact sheet with good statistics and information tends to be read, filed, and referred to again when needed.

Be Constructive.

If a bill deals with a problem you admit exists, but you believe that the bill is the wrong approach, tell the Member what you believe the right approach would be.

Be Persistent.

Do not stop with one contact. In many cases, you may want to write a letter, followed by a visit with the Member when he or she is home during a congressional recess, and then a telephone call to the Member immediately prior to a scheduled floor vote. Keep the pressure on the legislator.

Always Be Courteous. Do not Threaten.

It will get you nowhere — except perhaps investigated by the Federal Bureau of Investigation — to threaten a public official. State your case in a concise manner, be persistent, but never threaten.

Keep in Regular Contact.

Do not just write a letter or make a personal visit when you have a specific request for your legislator. Write a Member to congratulate him or her on a speech or to extend thanks for a recent vote. It is much easier to contact a Member directly, with a specific request, if you have established a regular relationship.

Report Back.

The most effective strategies involve coordination between you — the grassroots lobbyist — and your organization's lobbyists in Washington. Washington lobbyists often are told by Members, "I have received no mail on that issue, so I cannot support your position." If you receive a reply letter from a Member indicating support, that letter can used by the Washington lobbyist to ensure that Member's support. Also, Members want to hear from their constituents. If the Washington lobbyist can show copies of letters to the Member from his or her constituents, it is invaluable in prompting action by the Member.

Say 'Well Done'.

Members of Congress are human, too. They appreciate an occasional "thank you" from people who believe that they have done the right thing.

Letters

If only one lesson is learned from this entire manual, let it be: *your letter counts*. Do not underestimate the influence of a single letter. Occasionally, a well-crafted personal letter sent to your Member has enough impact that that Member reads the letter into the record of House or Senate floor debate. The letter is reprinted in the *Congressional Record* and subsequently read by other Members, their staffs, the press, and interested individuals. A journalist could use your letter as the basis of a column emphasizing the need for a certain bill to be enacted into law. That single letter could become the most influential factor in getting a bill passed into law. Farfetched? Not really. Most letters will not travel such a distinguished path, but some certainly have.

Remember, if appropriate, to use letterhead in your letter writing campaign — e.g., when you are representing a SNA or local district. In other cases, it may be more appropriate to use plain paper or stationery. In both cases, make sure your name and address are clearly printed on your letter.

Keep your letter to one page, if possible, and never exceed two pages, even if you are writing on a complex issue such as health care reform. Address your letter correctly as follows:

To a Senator:

The Honorable _____(NAME)_____
United States Senate
Washington, DC 20510

Dear Senator _____:

To a Representative:

The Honorable _____(NAME)_____
U.S. House of Representatives
Washington, DC 20515

Dear Representative _____:
  or
Dear Congressman/Congresswoman _____:

When writing to the chairman/chairwoman of a committee or the Speaker of the House, it is proper to address him or her as:

Dear Mr. Chairman or Madam Chairwoman or
Dear Mr./Madam Speaker

To establish your credibility immediately, begin your letter by identifying yourself, your connection to the legislation, and your profession:

"I am Jane Doe, RN, from Zoe, California, and a member of the California Nurses Association. In addition, I am employed by the Zoe Memorial Hospital as a staff nurse in the oncology unit. I am writing to you today about the need for mammography screening procedures."

Immediately, you have established yourself as:

1. a constituent;
2. a health care expert;
3. a member of a large organization; and,
4. a credible source on mammography.

Limit yourself to one issue per letter. A letter that addresses ten different subjects loses its effectiveness. It is better to send ten separate letters, each on a single subject. Include pertinent fact sheets, brochures, and short background materials. If the issue you are interested in is the subject of legislation that has been introduced, cite the bill number.

Include information on the local impact of a proposal, if possible. For example:

"The issue of lack of accessibility in the health-care delivery system is illustrated by the fact that five out of ten women in Zoe County do not receive prenatal care because of the lack of transportation facilities."

Ask for a response:

"I would appreciate hearing your views on this issue."

Establish yourself as a source of information:

"If you need any further information regarding this bill's effect on my hospital/town/(whatever), please feel free to contact me."

Although the central activity of each congressional office is answering constituent mail (Representatives receive hundreds of letters per week, senators hundreds per day.), some letters do go unanswered. Let your Member know that you expect a response. If you do not receive one in a reasonable amount of time, write again and indicate that you still are waiting.

The Form Letter

One of the most frequent questions asked about writing to Members of Congress is, how much of an impact does a form letter have. Members usually think form letters are computer-generated. They often will check if the signers of the form letters are constituents. However, if you are wavering between doing nothing or sending a form letter, then, by all means, send a form letter. If you are able to take an extra ten minutes to compose your own letter, its effectiveness will increase your communications exponentially.

Lobbying campaigns can involve constituents signing their own form letters. This is a useful method for breaking in new grassroots lobbyists. However, it is important to emphasize that the next step is writing your own letter. This rule does not preclude the use of model letters or sample letters in your group's efforts. New grassroots lobbyists often feel more comfortable using a sample letter as a prototype for writing their own. It is a good idea to alter the sample letter slightly by including a personal point of view or anecdote in each individual letter.

To Type or not to Type

Members often say that the only way to ensure that a personal letter is a personal letter these days is if it is handwritten — bad penmanship notwithstanding. In the old days, a letter typed on a portable typewriter was just as effective as a handwritten note. In some instances, a typed note was preferable because of illegible handwriting. This rule no longer applies. The fact that a computer can spit out 350 seemingly personal letters in a matter of minutes has made typed personal letters suspect.

Telephone Calls

Telephone calls to your Member are useful. They are effective primarily for obtaining information. If you want to know the number of a bill or how a Member voted, you can call either the Washington or the district office and talk to a staff member. If you are making a lobbying call, you should keep your message very short.

FIGURE 17

CONGRESSIONAL LETTER-WRITING TIPS

- State your reason for writing in the first paragraph. If your letter pertains to a specific piece of legislation, identify it by title and/or subject matter — i.e., House bill: H.R.___, Senate bill: S.___ .

- Be specific and include key information. Use examples to support your position whenever possible. Explain the importance of the issue or specific legislation.

- If you are writing to ask for co-sponsorship or a vote for or against a bill, say so. Tell your representative specifically what you would like him or her to do to be of assistance to your cause.

- Be brief but informative. Keep your letter to a maximum of two pages, and if possible, one page.

- Limit each letter to only one topic.

- In closing the letter, always offer your assistance — or your group's assistance — as a resource for more information.

- Thank your representative if he or she pleases you with a vote on an issue. Everyone appreciates a complimentary letter — and remembers it. On the other hand, if a vote is contrary to your position, do not hesitate to let him or her know in a polite manner. That will be remembered, too.

Generally, when you call a legislator's office, you will speak with a staffer rather than directly with the Member. Indicate the nature of your call and the person you would like to talk with — "I would like to speak to the person who handles health care issues." If that person is not in, whoever answers the phone will often tell you that staff person's name. Write it down and the next time you call, you can ask for that person. He or she is the person most likely to give you a clear indication of the Member's position on that issue. You can use this information in a follow-up letter.

Sometimes it is possible to schedule a telephone call with a Member in advance. Members often are receptive to having a conference call set up among themselves and several constituents to discuss a pressing issue.

If you do not know your Member's Washington office telephone number, call the Capitol switchboard at (202) 224-3121 or (202) 225-3121 and ask to be connected.

Telephone calls should only be used to deliver a quick message. They are not useful when a lot of substance or background material is necessary. Prior to major votes on the House and Senate floors, Members will receive large numbers of calls. Staffs keep a running tally of how many calls are "for" and how many calls are "against" a specific piece of legislation. If you want your representative or senator to vote "yes" on a certain bill, two telephone calls may not be very effective, but fifty will. Use this strategy if you have a lot of people you can depend on to participate in a telephone campaign.

Recently, both the question of whether to dispatch troops to the Persian Gulf and the nomination of Clarence Thomas to the Supreme Court resulted in thousands of calls to congressional offices. Prior to votes like these, Members ask their staffs for the results of tallies and may receive an answer such as, "150 for and 180 against." Although these calls may not change a Member's vote, they will give him or her an idea whether that vote does or does not represent the majority of his or her constituency.

It also is possible to call the White House and urge the president to sign a bill. Each day, the tally of phone calls is noted by an assistant to the president. For example, when the Department of Health and Human Services appropriations bill was sent to the president (with a provision reversing a regulation that prohibited health care professionals from providing abortion counseling at federally funded family-planning clinics), hundreds of individuals and organizations called the White House either urging the president to sign or to veto the bill.

Telegrams

Telegrams, just like telephone calls, should be utilized for the same quick message sent by a lot of individuals. Prior to a controversial vote, Members often receive a large number of telegrams urging them to cast a particular vote. To be effective, the telegrams must arrive in bulk and at critical points in the legislative process. Telegrams can be used to express a sense of urgency. For example, if a debate is taking place on the floor of the Senate and you want to express your opinion, you can pick up the telephone and have a telegram delivered to your senators within a few hours.

Telegrams and other forms of electronic communication, such as telexes, can be used to elicit general support — "Please support *Nursing's Agenda for Health Care Reform.*" But they are utilized more often for a specific vote — "Please vote yes on H.R. 1 when it is considered tomorrow." Include your name and address when sending your telegram so the Member can verify its authenticity.

Telegrams are useful vehicles for mobilizing your grassroots constituency. Western Union has developed messages — "Mailgrams" and "Personal Opinion Messages" — that are significantly less expensive than a personal telegram. Personal Opinion Messages can be used to write your own message to a Member on a specific issue. These types of telegrams are generally less expensive than regular telegrams and are sent directly to Congress.

As a leader of your grassroots effort, you can set up a telephone number with Western Union that can be used by your members. If they call this telephone number and ask for a predetermined operator, they only have to request that a telegram on the organization's issue be sent. You have agreed with Western Union that three different messages (which are automatically rotated) will be sent out with the person's name and address. In fact, the organizational member does not even have to identify his or her Member of Congress; the telegram operator will look it up.

This method is useful if you are trying to mobilize large numbers of people who will not sit down and write to their Members. The total cost to an organization's member to use a pre-selected message on a telegram is about $5.00. This method also is useful if you want to send out a flyer throughout your state urging people to call the Western Union number and have a telegram sent (e.g., a recent television advertisement, paid for by a national civil liberties organization, encouraged people to call a "900" number to send a "personal" telegram to Members of Congress regarding family planning).

In the past, Members used to pay a great deal of attention to telegrams, because studies showed that only very politically active constituents would pay for such a relatively expensive form of communication to deliver their messages quickly. But today, as the cost of sending electronic messages has decreased, the sense of importance regarding telegrams also has diminished.

Some Members have installed electronic mailboxes in their computer systems so constituents with compatible computers can send them quick messages. It is too soon to determine whether this is an effective communications vehicle.

Postcards

Postcards have much the same utility as the Western Union pre-selected messages. Although postcards' impact on Members' actions is less than the other methods already described, they can be used by your local grassroots campaign to mobilize people. For example, on broad social issues, Washington lobby groups often have thousands of postcards pre-printed with attention-grabbing logos and catchy statements so their combined organizational memberships simply have to sign their names and addresses and mail them to their Members. These postcards entice people who are not used to lobbying to express their opinions on a certain issue. And pre-printed postcards are extremely inexpensive to print.

Receiving a large number of postcards may not change a legislator's mind on an issue, but it will serve as an indication that many constituents share similar views. But, remember, unless you can count on a large number being sent to a Member's office, they are ineffective.

Petitions

The effectiveness of petitions in lobbying campaigns is very limited. Members are suspicious of whether the people who sign petitions are really who they say they are and are really constituents.

Petitions are more effective when it comes to public relations. For example, if you have 10,000 people sign a petition calling for better health care and you present this petition to the Speaker of the House on the steps of the Capitol, in front of representatives of major media outlets, you can almost guarantee your event will receive attention. With this strategy, though attention may be paid to your issue on the nightly news, the petition itself may do little to impress Members (hence, the story on the nightly news is a perfect example of indirect lobbying).

Testifying at Legislative Hearings

Testifying at public hearings is a very effective method of lobbying. If there is a field hearing at which you think your local organization or coalition should testify, prepare a written request to present testimony. Once that request is granted (you can always submit written testimony that will be included in the public record of the hearing if your request to present oral testimony is denied), prepare your testimony.

Your goal is to share your views on a legislative proposal with the Members of the committee, and, also, the media, and, through them, with the public, as well. If your request to testify is accepted, that acceptance probably was based either on the assumption that you represent a large number of people or that you have an expertise on the subject being discussed.

Find out what the hearing will be covering. Is it a broad topic (e.g., health care reform) or a specific piece of legislation? Never try to "wing it" at congressional hearings. You will need to prepare a written statement as well as a short summary of your written remarks. You may also want to prepare a one- or two-page press release on your testimony. All congressional committees will limit your oral statement to five minutes; however, you also may submit a written statement. Often, that written statement is not permitted to exceed ten pages. The committee will require at least fifty copies of your testimony forty-eight hours in advance of the hearing. It is important to adhere to these rules.

You should rehearse your oral statement to make certain it does not exceed five minutes. Read it aloud several times. Spend some time with your friends or colleagues answering anticipated questions.

During most congressional hearings, a witness may be accompanied by an attorney or technical expert. If you are representing the head of an association or coalition, you may wish to bring a technical expert with you. You would present the testimony as well as receive questions from the Members, but defer to your colleague to handle those questions which you cannot answer. If you are representing a coalition, be prepared to answer questions about the make-up of your coalition, its funding, and the number of member organizations.

When you arrive to testify, be prepared to wait. Although time limits are placed on witnesses' oral testimony, time constraints on Members' statements and questions are rarely adhered to and schedules often are delayed. This does not mean, however, that you should arrive late. If you are not present when your name is called to appear before the committee, your opportunity to present your testimony will be lost. It is a good idea to arrive early and listen to the witnesses who precede you. That way, you will know which Members are present and who among them is asking friendly or hostile questions. You also will be able to rebut previous witnesses' testimony if it conflicts with your own.

When you begin your remarks, you should request that your written statement be entered into the record and state that you will summarize your remarks. The chairman/chairwoman of the committee will respond, "So ordered." Address the committee Members as "Congressman" or "Congresswoman" and the chairman/chairwoman as "Mr. Chairman" or "Madam Chairwoman." Even if you are on a first name basis with a Member, this is not the time to display your friendship.

Do some research on the Members. Be familiar with who your supporters are and who your opponents may be so you can tailor your responses to questions, if necessary. Prior to the hearing, the committee staff are available to help you. Feel free to call upon them if you need any type of assistance. They may also provide you with information on the concerns of individual committee Members on a particular bill.

Don't lose your temper in front of the committee, and, by extension, the public. This will help neither your cause nor your reputation. Be prepared for interruptions — e.g., staff whispering to the Members, bells, and telephones. It is possible that the chairman/chairwoman as well as other Members may leave the room for a while and that you will be testifying before only one or two Members. Continue to do so, unless instructed otherwise. At the end of your testimony, thank the committee for the opportunity to present your statement.

Following your oral testimony, and that of the other witnesses on your panel, committee Members will ask questions. On occasion, committee staff will advise you ahead of time concerning questions that a Member may ask. Most of the time, however, you must be prepared to answer questions extemporaneously.

If you do not know the answer, do not lie. The Member may be testing your knowledge base. It is perfectly acceptable to answer a question with a reply that you do not know the answer, but you would be happy to submit it in writing. If time is running short, the Members may indicate that they will submit questions to you in writing that they would like you to answer.

The hearing record is open for ten days following the hearings. If you promised to submit additional materials, send those materials as soon as possible. A few weeks after your oral testimony, you will receive a transcript of your oral statement as recorded by the congressional hearing recorder. An accompanying letter will advise you that you may correct any mistakes, such as misspellings, but you may not change the substance of your remarks. You must return this transcript to the committee within ten days.

The Personal Visit

Personal visits with your senator or representative are a very effective means of grassroots lobbying; they often can lay the foundation for future contacts. They can take place in the Member's district office closest to your home or in the Washington office.

You can increase your chances of arranging a face-to-face meeting by involving representatives from several groups, thus increasing the meeting's attractiveness and importance to the Member. It may take some time to arrange a meeting with your Member. If he or she is unavailable, it still is useful to arrange a meeting with a staff member.

Making an Appointment

To schedule an appointment, call your Member's office and ask for the appointments secretary. If you are on good terms with another staff person, it may be useful to call that person to see if they will pave your way with the appointments secretary. This is a very important person in a congressional office; he or she has the most control over how the Member's time is allocated. If you want to arrange a meeting in the district, follow the same procedure. Call the district office and indicate that you (or your group) would like to schedule a meeting when the senator or representative is home during a recess.

In Washington, once you get through to the appointments secretary, tell him or her whom you represent and the subject you want to discuss. For example:

> "Hello, my name is Jane Doe and I will be in Washington during the week of February 14. I am a registered nurse with the Alabama Nurses Association and would like to meet with Senator Beaux on the issue of health care reform."

If the Member is not available, ask to meet with the staff person who handles the relevant issue. If it is to be a real working meeting, the time you spend with the staff person, who is the expert on the issue, may be more productive than a meeting with the legislator. If you plan to take additional people to the meeting, tell the appointments secretary how many people to expect (congressional offices do not like to be surprised with unexpected visitors).

You will probably be allowed about fifteen to thirty minutes for your appointment. Be sure to reconfirm the appointment as the time nears. Unexpected emergencies are a daily occurrence in Congress. If there is a vote on the floor before or during your meeting, you will have to wait while the Member goes to the House or Senate to cast his or her vote. Do not be offended; this is a common occurrence which often cannot be predicted.

Planning Your Appointment

If you are to be the leader of a group meeting with your Member, hold a planning session prior to your visit. Since you will have a short time with him or her, it is useful to have people assigned to address certain topics. Appoint a spokesperson who will call on other members of the group to speak.

For example, if you are meeting with your Member on the issue of pay equity, you may assign one person to talk about discrimination in job evaluation systems, a second to address successful state laws pertaining to pay equity, and a third to articulate the position of your SNA on pay equity. In this manner, each participant has an assigned role and the meeting is structured effectively.

Going to Your Appointment

Some of the suggestions offered below will ensure a smooth meeting with your legislator.

- Be on time for your appointment. If you are even five minutes late, the Member may have gone on with his or her next appointment, you will have started with a bad impression, and your opportunity may very well have been lost.

- Greet your legislator with a firm handshake, introduce yourself, and present your business card (if applicable; it also helps the Member remember names).

- Open the meeting with a comment to establish a tie between the legislator and yourself — e.g., a discussion of mutual friends, common interests in the state, a thank you for a recent hearing, vote, or floor speech.

- Next, if appropriate, state how many of the Member's constituents you represent and what your mission is. Identify the subject of the meeting and present your facts in an orderly fashion. Talk about a specific bill, its status, and action you would like the legislator to take. Use your own background and experience to explain your request.

  > "I am a nurse from an inner city hospital in New York. I have seen in my work that the ability to be directly reimbursed by Medicaid would increase access to health care for a population in need. I urge you to co-sponsor S. 1842," or,

  > "As a nurse, I am in the front lines of the health-care delivery system. I am asking you to support comprehensive health care reform, because I see the results of the lack of access for people in this country."

- Use personal anecdotes and statistics when appropriate. Keep to your schedule. Do not go off on a tangent, wasting valuable time. Realize that you may be interrupted by the Member's staff during the meeting, especially if a vote comes up on the floor (see section on *Legislative Bells and Signals,* p. 82).

- Because opportunities for personal meetings with the Member are limited, you should always ask for the name of the staff person who handles your issue and indicate that you would like to follow-up with him or her. It is possible that the legislator will ask that staff person to attend the meeting.

- Be succinct. This may be the most important issue in the world to you, but it is only one of several dozen on your legislator's plate. If you start to ramble on, you will lose your audience in a very short time.

- Also, do not become too technical in the examples and background materials you use to justify your position. You may be an expert on this subject, but chances are the legislator is not. If you lapse into technical jargon, you will lose him or her. Remember — the impression you make in a fifteen-minute meeting could last for years.

- Leave a one- or two-page fact sheet with the Member, summarizing the issue and your position(s), along with the names and telephone numbers of contact people (if the Member should wish to obtain further information).

- As you conclude the meeting, thank the Member for his or her time. Do not dawdle. In all likelihood, the Member has another meeting scheduled immediately after you leave.

- Follow up after the meeting with a letter thanking the Member, reiterating your position, and including any information requested during the meeting. If the legislator or staff person should ask for additional materials, respond quickly. By establishing yourself as a reliable source of information, you will improve your access to your Member.

Another way to meet your legislator is to invite him or her to address a particular audience, or to answer questions (which often requires less preparation than a speech). As a leader in a community group, a hospital, or a local organization, you can play host to that Member. Members are receptive to visiting places where they can meet with large numbers of constituents (e.g., a hospital cafeteria). They also like to attend business and union meetings. To set up this type of appointment, call either the appointments secretary in the Washington office or the constituent-services staff member in the district office. Generally, these events need to be scheduled months in advance. Be flexible about the dates and try for a time during a recess.

STEP-BY-STEP GRASSROOTS LOBBYING STRATEGY GUIDE

During each step of the legislative and regulatory process, there are specific strategies that are particularly effective and that should be incorporated into your grassroots's mobilization effort. These are discussed below.

Introduction of Legislation

The first strategy is to define your mission in clear and precise terms. If your goal is the provision of direct reimbursement for advanced practice nurses under Medicare, you must first define how to accomplish that goal. Convene a meeting of technical experts (e.g., nurse practitioners and clinical nurse specialists) and legislative and political experts to map out your general strategies. Form a coalition of individuals and organizations pursuing the same goal.

After you have determined your goal, identify a legislator (in this case, a Member of Congress) who would be willing to introduce the legislation. Schedule a meeting with his or her staff to work out the broad agenda and follow it up with a meeting with the Member to request his or her sponsorship of the bill. Assist the Member's staff with the drafting of the bill (especially with definitions and the scope of the legislation) to make sure that your interests are represented. You will want to provide the Member's staff with information on the history of reimbursement to nurses, statistics on the impact of reimbursement on health care, and the political feasibility of implementing such a proposal. It often is useful to identify a Member in each chamber of Congress and have the representative and the senator introduce companion measures. Be sure that the staff people of both offices work together in the drafting of the legislation.

You will want to convince other Members to co-sponsor the bill, showing support for the legislation when it is introduced in the House and Senate. Often, the primary sponsor will write a "Dear Colleague" to other Members to encourage them to become co-sponsors. Then, when a bill is introduced, it lists both the sponsor and co-sponsors.

While it is important to have a large number of co-sponsors, it also is very effective to have a variety of co-sponsors, thus showing bipartisan support. You always want the Members of the committee to which the bill will be referred as co-sponsors. If a Member is listed as a co-sponsor, it is assumed that he or she supports the bill and will facilitate the bill's progress through the committee. If possible, it also is important to gain the support of the leadership for your proposal.

Co-sponsor strategies vary depending upon the primary sponsor and the type of legislation. When the Family and Medical Leave Act was introduced, even though there were over 150 co-sponsors, great efforts were made to influence southern Democrats to become co-sponsors because, by and large, they support moderate social policies. In addition, there was a reaching out to new Members, who may not be as knowledgeable about a particular legislative proposal as their more senior colleagues.

On occasion, you may not want a Member to co-sponsor a bill immediately upon introduction. For example, you may ask a very liberal Member to refrain from co-sponsorship until the bill has progressed through the committee stage, because moderate and conservative members may shy away from co-sponsoring a proposal when a liberal's name appears on the legislation.

After the bill is introduced, it is time to map out additional strategies. Before asking other Members for support, it is useful to have developed your one-page fact sheet detailing the content and impact of the proposed legislation. This information can prove invaluable in convincing a Member to support a bill. You may want to expand your coalition to include other interested groups. Also at this point, you should initiate your first letter writing campaign urging other Members to co-sponsor your bill.

If a bill was introduced that addresses your concerns , but is not the proposal that will meet your needs, you will have to decide on one of two courses: how to amend the bill to better suit what you want or how to defeat the bill if it has a negative impact on your cause. Comprehensive strategies include not only enacting a bill into law, but, also, amending legislative proposals. Often, several different versions of the same proposal will be introduced. It is your responsibility as a grassroots lobbyist to determine which bill you like best and how to promote that version. Always anticipate opposition to any legislative proposal.

Committee Consideration of Legislation

Probably no single part of the legislative process plays a more important role in influencing legislation than the hearing process. After a bill is introduced and referred to committee, the first hurdle is to get a public hearing. Write to all committee Members (or sub-committee, if appropriate) to emphasize the importance of the bill and the need for a hearing.

Your letter writing skills become critical at this point. This is the time to explain in detail the need for the legislation and its potential benefits to various constituencies. If you have a network of supporters that extends beyond your community or state, urge them to write too.

If a hearing is held on the bill, ask to submit either oral or written testimony. If your resources permit, testifying at a congressional hearing is an invaluable experience.

After the hearings, it is important to monitor the mark-up session. The committee will schedule at least one session of debate on the proposal with the opportunity for all committee Members to amend it. If a Member of the committee is planning to attach weakening amendments to your proposal, you should write to each Member explaining why they are harmful.

Letter writing skills are again important once a bill is scheduled to be voted on in committee. Although, generally, letters are a useful vehicle only in addressing your Member, this is the one exception. You are speaking to the committee Members, not as a constituent, but as an expert in your specialty. For example, you may want to explain why the Nurse Education Act must be re-authorized with higher funding levels in order to increase the number of certified non-physician practitioners in rural areas.

Even though your Member does not sit on the subcommittee or committee considering the legislation, it still is useful to write and express your views to him or her. Members often testify at hearings. Urge yours to testify or to contact his or her colleagues who serve on the committee with jurisdiction.

While the first step is getting the bill considered by committee, the second is to get an acceptable version passed by the committee. It is easy to kill a bill in committee. One Member can offer enough weakening amendments to change the very nature of the bill and make the legislation's intent disappear.

Be prepared to act quickly on proposed amendments. A Member may decide the night prior to the committee mark-up session that he or she will offer an amendment. That Member will lobby other Members of the committee to determine whether they will support the amendment. If you are working with a coalition, you may need to call a meeting of your group to determine if you can "live with" the amendment. The committee process forces Members, as well as constituents, to compromise on their original proposals. Determine which compromises are acceptable and which are unacceptable. Stick with your choices.

A bill may go through several committees if it covers a broad subject area (e.g., health care reform). In such cases, you may choose to focus your lobbying efforts on one of the committees where you have the most influence. For example, if your representative is the chairman/chairwoman of a subcommittee of the House Energy and Commerce Committee, your efforts would be better concentrated in that arena than in the Ways and Means Committee. It is possible for two committees to mark up the same bill differently. A bill can take on many different forms between introduction and final passage.

After a bill has been approved by a committee, the committee staff writes a report that describes the purpose and scope of the bill, explains any amendments, and includes cost estimates for implementation of the legislation. Committee Members opposed to all or part of the bill may submit written dissenting views for incorporation into the report.

Report language can establish legislative intent. For example, many appropriations bills set out only the amount of money an agency or department might spend, while the accompanying committee report contains directives on how Congress expects the money to be spent. Language often is included in the committee report but not in the bill. In a recent appropriations measure, increased funding was provided for the National Cancer Institute. Although the bill itself did not stipulate the exact manner in which those funds were to be expended, the report language indicated that the funds should be spent on breast and cervical cancer research. It has become common practice for committees — including House and Senate conference committees — to include instructions in their reports on how government agencies should interpret and enforce the law. The courts often have relied on these guidelines.

Lobbyists can influence the writing of the committee report. It is useful to include statements in the committee report that could not be included in the actual legislation. This type of lobbying is aided by a working relationship with the committee staff so you may suggest report language at the appropriate time.

Press strategies also are useful during committee consideration of a bill (See **How To Handle the Press**, p.110). "Op-Ed" pieces in relevant committee Members' local newspapers will be read by Members and may influence how they vote on a certain bill.

Rules Committee Action

In the House, after a bill has been reported out of committee, it goes to the Rules Committee for a decision on the type of debate that will take place on the floor. As a grassroots lobbyist, you can lobby for the most advantageous rule.

The majority of legislation is considered under an *open rule*, permitting amendments. A *modified open rule* means that only certain sections of a bill — as determined by the Rules Committee — are open to amendment. In certain cases, legislation is considered under a *closed rule*. This means that a bill cannot be subject to any floor amendments. A tax bill, for example, generally is considered under a closed rule in the House. If this is not done, there would be countless floor amendments which would seriously jeopardize the carefully crafted revenue balance achieved with the provisions of the original bill. A strategy to defeat legislation is to propose weakening amendments. However, if a bill is considered under a closed rule, this possibility is eliminated.

Floor Lobbying

Lobbying when a bill goes to the floor of the House or Senate for a vote is slightly different from lobbying up to this point. When the full House or Senate is voting on the bill, your only important contact is your own representative or senators. You now are lobbying as a constituent rather than on behalf of a large group.

Your message should be short and to the point. This is the time to use postcards, telegrams, and telephone calls. Concentrate on generating short notes in great quantities. Usually the vote will consist of one or two amendments — often including a substitute amendment by the opposing side — and then the final vote.

Your message should be short and clear:

"Vote for H.R. 3 without any weakening amendments."

An effective strategy to use during floor votes is to develop a *swing list*. It is difficult to lobby all 435 Members of the House. Develop a list containing five columns of information. The first column, "Definite Yes," includes Members who have co-sponsored the legislation as well as those who have written to their constituents promising their support. The second column, "Definite No," includes those Members who have indicated that there is no way they will support the proposal. Write to the definite "yeses" to firm up their votes. Do not waste your time on the definite "noes."

The remaining three columns should consist of a "Leaning Yes" column, a "Leaning No" column, and an "Undecided" column. Members listed in these columns should receive concentrated lobbying. These Members are your swing list. This is a very useful tool for coalition lobbying; people will know where to concentrate their efforts. It is important, however, that you insist that your swing list remain confidential. You do not want either Members or the press to see your working strategy. Keep your list flexible so that Members can move from "Undecided" to "Leaning Yes," but be sure of their positions prior to moving them to a "Definite Yes" or "Definite No" category.

Conference Committee Strategies

If the House and Senate pass similar bills that contain some differences, a conference committee must meet to work those out. It is essential that you follow the proceedings of a conference committee to determine the final outcome of your legislation.

To lobby the conference committee, you must first determine which version you support — the House or Senate. It is possible to support one provision in a House-passed bill and another provision in the Senate-passed bill. Often, a combination of the House and Senate bills may be the best alternative. You can lobby your own representative or senators to, in turn, lobby the conference committee Members. Or, you can write directly to the conference committee Members.

There are times that conference committee proceedings are resistant to lobbying efforts. If a compromise is carefully crafted so it will pass both chambers quickly and easily, the Members of the conference committee may have little interest in what you have to say.

Return to the House and Senate Floors

After the conference committee has reconciled the two versions of a bill and combined them into one, that bill must return to the House and Senate floors for final passage. This procedure usually is just a formality in which no lobbying strategies are necessary.

Presidential Signature Strategies

Although it is difficult to have any impact on the actions of the White House, you can write the president or call the White House ([202]456-1414) and leave a message urging the president either to sign or veto a bill.

Overriding a Veto

If the president vetoes a bill, it sometimes is returned to the Congress for an attempt to override the veto. Overriding a presidential veto is difficult because it requires a two-thirds vote of the membership of each chamber.

Lobbying strategies for a veto override are similar to floor strategies, except the message is shorter. Lobby either to sustain the veto or override it. No amendments are allowed during a veto override vote. It is especially important to firm up your "Leaning Yes" votes. Sometimes Members who voted for the original bill will switch positions if they are of the same political party as the president because their loyalty to the president overshadows their concerns about the bill under consideration. Be aware of these situations.

Regulatory Lobbying

After a bill has passed Congress and been signed into law by the president, it is referred to the federal agency of jurisdiction so that implementing regulations can be written. Implementing regulations can destroy a good law as well as limit the implementation of a new law. There are opportunities to influence regulations both before and after they are finalized.

Identify and establish contact with those agency officials who are considered the "in-house experts" in certain issue areas. Get to know these people through informational meetings prior to the time when you will need to lobby them. Usually, these people are overworked, underpaid federal employees who will welcome any help you can give them. As a lobbyist, make it your job to provide these officials with information when needed.

After a proposed rule is published, there is a time period during which the general public can submit comments on that rule. This process usually is open. You can submit your own comments and read the comments submitted by other organizations and individuals. Sometimes the agency will hold an information hearing on the regulations being considered. In this case, you can request to present your case at the hearing.

After the comment period, the agency will publish its final rule. If the rule still does not fit your agenda, you will have to return to Congress to alter the regulations through legislation. If the final rule does meet with your approval, you will have to continue to monitor the agency's actions to ensure that they enforce the regulations. Request to be placed on an agency's mailing list. When the agency publishes notices and press releases concerning regulations, you will receive them.

It is useful for grassroots lobbyists to keep Members of Congress and relevant congressional committees apprised of federal agencies' actions. If a federal agency does not adhere to congressional intent, Congress can exert pressure on that agency (e.g., by calling for oversight hearings).

You can influence agencies indirectly through the nominations and appropriations processes. As a constituent, you can lobby Congress on political appointments to federal agencies, influencing the process that determines which people are placed in policy making positions in the federal government. By lobbying for political appointments, you can place "friends" in positions where they will formulate policy in line with your philosophy. For example, after the 1992 presidential election, ANA instituted the ANA Appointments Project to identify nurses, with excellent academic and political credentials, to recommend for some of the more than 3,500 full-time federal government positions filled by persons appointed by the president.

You also can lobby Congress to increase or decrease the appropriations for a federal agency. For example, in recent years, many groups have criticized the U.S. Commission on Civil Rights for not fulfilling its obligation to enforce civil rights statutes in this country. In response, Congress has appropriated fewer dollars for shorter time periods until such time as the Commission fulfills its mandate. Another example is the newly created Office of Women's Health Research at the National Institutes of Health (NIH). The administration proposed $1.5 million for its initial start-up budget. Women's health advocates successfully lobbied for a $10 million budget for this new office, believing that the administration should place a greater emphasis on women's health research.

Legislative Status Reports

It is imperative that, as a grassroots lobbyist, you keep track of the legislative records of your Member(s). This information should include the biographical material you have collected, letters written by as well as received from your representatives and senators, newspaper stories, staff contact names and phone numbers, and the key votes cast during a session of Congress. In this manner, you will begin to develop your own *Congressional Profile*. This information will prove to be an invaluable resource as you develop and maintain your legislative contacts.

GETTING TO, FROM, AND AROUND CAPITOL HILL

Capitol Hill ("the Hill") is the highest point in the District of Columbia. In addition to its blocks of residential neighborhoods and small businesses, it consists of the actual Capitol Building, five House of Representatives office buildings, three Senate office buildings, the Supreme Court, and three buildings for the Library of Congress (the Jefferson, Madison, and Adams buildings).

The Capitol Building and its immediate grounds are the point at which the city of Washington is divided into four quadrants — Northeast (NE), Northwest (NW), Southeast (SE), and Southwest (SW) — by East Capitol Street (which runs east/west), and South Capitol Street and North Capitol Street (which run north/south). Every street address in Washington (with the exception of East Cap-itol, South Capitol and North Capitol) is followed by the abbreviation for the quadrant in which it lies (e.g., First Street, NE, First Street, NW).

The actual layout of the Capitol is symmetrical with the Senate chamber on one side and the House chamber on the other. The north side of the Capitol houses the Senate chamber. Surrounding Senate office buildings, separate from the Capitol, are half a block north of it. The House office buildings are the same distance south of the House side of the Capitol (with the exception of the two annexes, which are slightly farther south).
(See Figure 18).

The Buildings

House

The offices of the 435 members of the House of Representatives are located in three office buildings along Independence Avenue, SE. Committee offices and staffs also are housed in these buildings as well as in two nearby buildings.

Following is a description of the House office buildings:

- *Cannon House Office Building (CHOB);* Independence Avenue and First Street, SE. Room numbers have three digits; the first digit indicates which floor.

- *Longworth House Office Building (LHOB)*; Independence and New Jersey Avenues, SE. Room numbers have four digits. The first digit (a "1") indicates the Longworth Building, the second digit indicates which floor in Longworth.

FIGURE 18

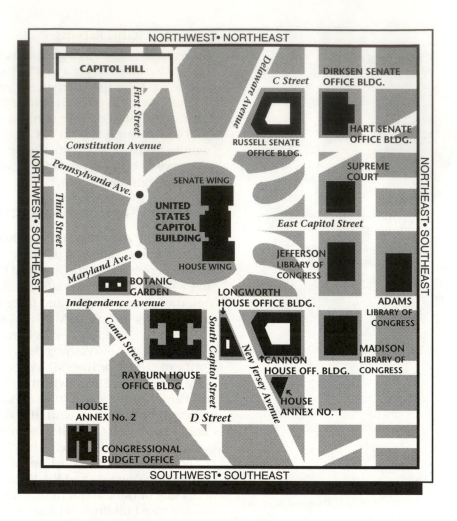

- *Rayburn House Office Building (RHOB);* Independence Avenue between First Street, SW and South Capitol Street. Room numbers have four digits. The first digit (a "2") indicates Rayburn Building, the second digit indicates which floor in Rayburn.

- *O'Neill House Office Building (OHOB or House Annex #1);* New Jersey Avenue and C Street, SE. Room numbers have three digits; first digit is the floor number.

- *Ford House Office Building (FHOB or House Annex #2);* 2nd and D Streets, SW. Room numbers have three digits; first digit is the floor number.

Senate

The three Senate office buildings are located along Constitution Avenue, NE. The offices of the 100 senators, as well as Senate committees, are located in these buildings.

- *Hart Senate Office Building (HSOB);* Constitution Avenue and 2nd Street, NE. Room numbers have three digits; first digit is the floor number.

- *Dirksen Senate Office Building (DSOB);* Constitution Avenue and First Street, NE. Room numbers have three digits; first digit is the floor number.

- *Russell Senate Office Building (RSOB);* Constitution and Delaware Avenues, NE. Room numbers have three digits; first digit is the floor number.

Visitor Access

Visitors can enter the House and Senate office buildings and the Capitol through entrances marked "Visitors' Entrances." Each building has entrances and facilities to accommodate physically disabled persons. Immediately inside is a security system similar to those in airports. Capitol police officers (Congress has its own relatively small police force, the U.S. Capitol Police.) inspect packages, bags, and purses before each person passes through a metal detector. Once inside, the visitor is free to visit Members' offices, attend open committee meetings, or watch the House and Senate floor proceedings.

To move from one building to another, visitors can go outside or use a series of pedestrian tunnels that connect House and Senate office buildings to the Capitol, and a separate internal subway that runs, on the House side, from the Rayburn Building to the Capitol, and on the Senate side, from each of the three Senate office buildings to the Capitol. There is no charge for the use of these subways. However, during votes on the House and Senate floors, only Members are allowed to use them. Unless you like to explore, it is far easier to walk outside.

Capitol police officers are stationed throughout the House and Senate office buildings and the Capitol building and are always willing to assist anyone needing directions or other information.

Attendance at Committee Hearings

Congressional committee hearings are held in the House and Senate office buildings as well as the Capitol.

A column entitled "Today in Congress" appears in the front section of the *Washington Post* each day that the House and/or Senate are in session. It provides a list of the committees and subcommittees meeting that day, subject(s) to be discussed, and the time and location of the meetings. The times that the House and Senate will convene on that day also are listed. Unless otherwise indicated, committee and subcommittee meetings and hearings are open to the public and require no pass to gain admission.

When Congress is in session, most committee hearings occur on Tuesdays, Wednesdays, and Thursdays.

For hearings on controversial, popular topics, plan to arrive at least an hour early to wait in line. Seats — and sometimes standing room — at such events are highly prized.

Admission to the House and Senate Galleries

The House and Senate galleries are located on the third floor of the Capitol. To observe floor proceedings in the House or Senate, a visitor must obtain gallery passes from his or her representative or senator (Both have passes for both chambers.). Without a current pass, admission to the visitors' galleries is prohibited.

Some rules to observe during gallery attendance: Any writing is forbidden; packages, bundles, cameras, suitcases, or briefcases are also prohibited and must be checked before entering the galleries. Also not allowed: standing or sitting in the doorways or aisles; smoking, eating or drinking, applauding, reading, taking photographs, and men wearing hats, except those worn for religious purposes. Children under six years of age are not permitted in the galleries.

Legislative Bells and Signals

When the House and Senate are in session, a series of lights and bells can be seen and heard in all of the office buildings and the Capitol to alert Members to specific legislative activities. A system of lights is built around most of the clocks in the House and Senate office buildings. It is useful to know what some of the flashing lights and ringing bells signify.

Senate

In the Senate, there is one long ring at the hour of convening. One red light on the right-hand side of the clocks remains lighted while the Senate is in session. Where lights exist (on most clocks in the Senate office buildings), they will correspond with the following bells:

1 Bell / 1 Light:	Yeas and Nays vote
2 Bells/2 Lights:	Quorum call
3 Bells/3 Lights:	Call of absentees
4 Bells/4 Lights:	Adjournment or Recess
5 Bells/5 Lights:	Five minutes remaining on yeas and nays vote
6 Bells/6 Lights:	Morning business concluded or temporary recess

House

In the House, there is one long ring at the hour of convening (this is preceded by three short rings fifteen minutes before convening).

When the House is in session, one red light on most clocks in the House office buildings remains lit. Where lights exist, they will correspond with the following bells:

1 Bell /1 Light:	Teller vote (not a recorded vote)
1 Long Bell /1 Light (Pause) followed by 3 bells /3 lights:	Start or continuation of a notice quorum call (this will be terminated if and when 100 Members appear)
1 Long Bell/1 Light:	Termination of a notice quorum call
2 Bells/2 Lights:	Yeas and Nays electronically recorded vote

2 Bells/2 Lights (Pause) followed by **2 Bells/2 Lights:**	Manual (as opposed to electronic) roll call vote. The bells are sounded again when the clerk reaches the letter "R."
2 Bells/2 Lights (Pause) followed by **5 Bells:**	First vote under suspension of the rules or on *clustered votes* (i.e., a number of votes taken in quick succession) (2 bells will ring five minutes later). The first vote will take fifteen minutes with successive votes at intervals of not less than five minutes. Each successive vote will be signaled by 5 bells.
3 Bells/3 Lights:	Regular quorum call (bells are repeated 5 minutes after the first ring)
4 Bells/4 Lights:	Adjournment of the House
5 Bells/5 Lights:	Five-minute electronically recorded vote
6 Bells/6 Lights:	Recess of the House

Transportation

Public parking spaces are a rare commodity on Capitol Hill. There is limited metered parking and most of the available on-street parking spaces are reserved for congressional staff during normal business hours. Public parking garages are expensive and, for the most part, are a considerable distance from the Capitol as well as the House and Senate office buildings.

It is a good idea to leave your car at home and either take a taxi or use Washington's subway system (known as the "Metro"). Cab fares in the city are not metered, but are determined by zones. Fares are higher during rush hour and with each additional passenger.

The Metro

The Metro is a safe, convenient, and cost-effective means of transportation in Washington. Dark brown metal columns with a large white "M" indicate Metro station entrances. The two stations closest to Capitol Hill are Capitol South (Blue and Orange subway lines) on the House side of the Hill and Union Station (Red line) on the Senate side.

Metro fares vary according to distance traveled and time of day (i.e., rush hour fares are higher than non-rush-hour fares). Fares can be determined by consulting the route and fare maps posted at all Metro stations. The current base fare is $1.00.

Subway travelers must purchase a "farecard" to enter and then exit the system. Each person over the age of five years must have one. Farecard vending machines are located in every Metro station. Request assistance from the attendant working in the station kiosk.

The Metro operates on a regular basis, seven days a week (5:30 a.m. to midnight) on weekdays; 8:00 a.m. until midnight on Saturdays, and 10:00 a.m. until midnight on Sundays. Schedules vary on holidays. To obtain information regarding Metro fares and schedules, call (202) 637-7000 from 6:00 a.m. to 11:30 p.m., seven days a week.

CHAPTER IV

COALITIONS

A *coalition* involves bringing together diverse groups, organizations, and/or individuals for a specific purpose. That purpose can vary from a legislative effort to pass a bill to organizing a political campaign to elect a nurse to Congress; from initiating a voter registration drive, to completing a community project, or establishing a collective bargaining unit.

Why form a coalition? The answer is simple — it makes any job easier. The strength of a coalition lies in the fact that each group, organization, or individual makes a contribution, whether it be in the form of people power, money, services, information, an endorsement, or contacts. To get a bill through a state assembly is a major undertaking. To share that goal and the work involved with other groups allows individuals to accomplish tasks in digestible chunks. "There is strength in numbers" is an old adage that works well in grassroots-lobbying coalition building.

Coalitions are very difficult to establish and maintain, but they are very effective mechanisms for lobbying or running a political campaign. As federal, state, and local governments have expanded, coalitions have become essential grassroots tools.

ESTABLISHING A COALITION

Forming a coalition requires planning. The first step is determining what type coalition best fits your needs. Coalitions can form to accomplish a single goal — such as passing a bill through Congress — or they can take on broader, multi-purpose causes such as improving long-term health care.

In addition to the type of coalition, examine what size coalition you want to build. A coalition needs to be large enough to have an impact, but small enough that the group can be controlled. Do you want to let the whole world join you in your efforts, or do you want to limit participation? Coalitions can be comprised of a board of experts or they can include every health and social welfare organization in the state.

When you invite an individual or an organization to join your coalition, they will want to know what you expect of them. Do you want them to lend their name or endorse a set of principles established by the coalition? How active will their participation be?

You should be prepared to brief potential members on the goals of the coalition, the tactics and strategies to be used to achieve those goals, general time lines for reaching the goals, and the role each organization will play. Informal coalition structures often begin with members promising to undertake specific tasks on an ongoing basis to support the coalition. As the coalition becomes more active, it may become more formal, hiring a staff to carry out its mission. Since that staff is working on behalf of all the members, it becomes necessary for the groups involved with the coalition to contribute predetermined levels of funds or services (e.g., membership fees).

After you have identified the type and size of the coalition, the next step is to target other like-minded groups and individuals in the community to join your efforts. Potential member organizations include: health organizations, women's groups, social workers, senior citizen advocates, community action alliances, mental health associations, disability groups, labor unions, medical associations and, on occasion, insurance and business organizations.

Prior to requesting the participation of any group, do a background check. Find out who the leaders of the organization are, and what other coalitions they belong to; determine the level of their influence in the community, and review their primary focus and agenda. In addition, try to ascertain what their motivation would be in joining your coalition. It is necessary to identify potential points of conflict before agreeing to a relationship among several organizations. Estimate what the prospective organization gains from belonging to the coalition as well as what strengths and weaknesses it contributes.

Because you started the coalition, you and your association are immediately established as a leader. For the coalition to always deliver a unified, consistent message, it is essential that a designated spokesperson be assigned to articulate the views and goals of the coalition to the media and general public. At this point, you must consider whether it is "political" for nurses to be at the forefront of the coalition. In most cases, it will be. The visibility gained by leading a coalition is invaluable. However, if the cause is one in which nurses may be viewed as self-serving, it is better to designate a member of another group as the spokesperson.

WORKING WITH A COALITION

At your first coalition meeting, the development of the agenda should be the primary focus. Be very clear on the coalition's positions. Insist on uniformity and consensus. Encourage the coalition members to be flexible and open-minded. It is important for participating organizations to be able to listen to other perspectives on any issue and be willing to compromise. If a point is in disagreement, drop it. It is better to agree to disagree on a point and exclude it from your agenda in the privacy of coalition meetings, prior to releasing your agenda publicly. You are bringing groups together for collective action. To gain and maintain political impact, it is essential to present a united front.

Avoid unnecessary conflicts between coalition members by keeping the agenda, as well as subsequent coalition activities, focused on your common goals. Do not let the coalition become an arena for conflicts over unrelated issues.

The next step is to plan the strategies with which the coalition will accomplish its goals. Assess your members' commitment — how many people do you have available to work. Make assignments based on people's strengths and talents. Also, assess your resources in terms of money and in-kind services. Do you have access to computers, printers, graphic artists, and copying machines? These are useful in a public education campaign.

Small task forces made up of coalition members are useful vehicles for dividing up the work. For example, in a legislative effort, task forces can be formed to deal with grassroots mobilization efforts, direct lobbying in the state capital, and media outreach. Coalition members serve on the task force that takes best advantage of their skills, contacts, and resources. It is important that all coalition members come together periodically to review strategies, coordinate activities, and assess the coalition's progress.

If you are a member of a coalition and would like to establish yourself in a leadership position, any contributions you can make in terms of human resources will enhance your opportunities. You also can donate money, provide the coalition with a meeting place, or lend your computer skills to maintaining the mailing list. Any of these activities will establish you as an essential player.

If you are the leader of the coalition, the responsibility for accomplishing all the tasks will lie with you. This is a very time-consuming position. Make sure you have people you can count on to complete their assignments. Do not overwork your members. Distribute the work equitably. Try to keep each individual and organization involved to its maximum potential. Recognize each member's contribution within the coalition in a public manner.

Establish an internal damage-control mechanism. Be aware that some coalition member organizations may have "hidden agendas" to benefit their own interests which may interfere with work toward the overall goal of the coalition. Try to identify these interests early in your coalition efforts, and, wherever possible, avoid public conflict. A recent example of such a situation was during debate on child care legislation, where groups advocating a comprehensive child-care bill found themselves in disagreement over the funding mechanism for the program. Some groups wanted vouchers that parents could use to pay for child care and other groups lobbied for grants to individual states to establish child care facilities. This conflict was recognized and instead of allowing it to evolve into a public battle, the coalition agreed on a combination of financing mechanisms for child care.

Finally, know when to stop. There is nothing more purposeless than a coalition that has outlived its effectiveness. The most obvious time to disband is after you have reached your goal, but this is not always what happens. At every step, assess your resources. There may come a time when your members are burned out. Some issues and goals may take years to accomplish, and a coalition's usefulness may decline as the years go by. If internal conflicts consume the coalition, it also is time to stop.

FIGURE 19

COALITION CHECKLIST

- **DETERMINE TYPE OF COALITION**
- **FORM COALITION**
- **PLAN AN AGENDA**
- **DETERMINE STRATEGIES**
- **MAKE ASSIGNMENTS AND FORM TASK FORCES**
- **DISBAND COALITION WHEN APPROPRIATE**

CHAPTER V

POLITICAL ACTION COMMITTEES*

"BEFORE YOU CAN BECOME
A STATESMAN, YOU FIRST HAVE
TO GET ELECTED, AND TO GET
ELECTED YOU HAVE TO BE
A POLITICIAN PLEDGING
SUPPORT FOR WHAT THE
VOTERS WANT."

Margaret Chase Smith
*First woman elected to both
the House and the Senate*

Political action committees (PACs) have become an integral part of the legislative and political process and significant vehicles for financing campaigns. From 1974 to 1990, the number of PACs increased from 608 to 4,172, and their numbers continue to grow.

PACS usually are created by existing organizations as a separate fund or entity. These funds finance campaigns for political office and educate their members on how to become involved in the political process. A few PACS are organized around specific issues with no organizational backing (e.g., Voters for Choice), but this tends to be the exception rather than the rule.

Federal election guidelines dictate how PACs are administered. PAC donations may be solicited only for the purpose of funding the campaigns of political candidates. However, an organization's general treasury funds may be used to support its political education efforts — such as voter registration programs — and the administrative costs of a PAC. For example, the ANA can fund a political education program, but the ANA PAC must solicit its own funds from the ANA membership to support political campaigns.

PAC campaign support for congressional candidates serves several important functions. It often will induce a representative or senator to back the organization's legislative interests on Capitol Hill, and it will help to insure that Members sympathetic to the group's goals will remain in office. In addition, a PAC often can secure access to a legislator for lobbyists who might not otherwise have such access. This, in turn, allows lobbyists the opportunity to present their case directly to the elected official.

No individual or group needs to tell a Member outright that future political support or opposition — as well as campaign contributions and campaign participation — hinge on how he or she votes on a particular bill, or whether he or she eventually responds favorably to the group and its legislative agenda. The legislator understands this without being told. He or she is well aware that when a group has a strong interest in a particular bill, support for that measure will win the group's friendship and approval, whereas a vote against it will insure the group's opposition.

---

* Portions of this chapter have been adapted from *The American Nurses Association Political and Legislative Handbook*. 1990. Washington, DC: American Nurses Association.

With the average campaign for a seat in the Senate costing more than $1.5 million and some races for the House of Representatives breaking the $1 million mark, candidates often need more than love, they need money. While corporations have been prohibited from making direct contributions to campaigns for federal office since 1907, and labor unions since 1943, their employees and members can form PACs, which then channel their contributions to particular candidates.

Trade associations and membership groups also give money to candidates through PACs. Though individuals, of course, can always contribute to candidates, organizations can earn more institutional credit if their members pool their resources, and, through PACs, make collective contributions to the candidates of their choice. In 1990, House and Senate candidates received $150.6 million from PACs, and PAC donations accounted for 38 percent of campaign funding for House candidates and 22 percent for Senate candidates.

Nurses have political power — in terms of numbers and knowledge. In recent years, tens of thousands of nurses across the country have become involved in the political process. These nurses have given hundreds of thousands of volunteer hours working for political candidates, have contributed funds to election campaigns, and have run for office themselves.

In purely political terms, nurses are making great strides as they move into leadership positions at all levels of government. Less than a decade ago, there were no nurses in any state legislature. Currently, over fifty nurses serve in elected positions at the state level. One nurse currently serves in Congress — Eddie Bernice Johnson (D-TX), first elected to the 103rd Congress.

THE ANA PAC

In the late 1960s, nurses throughout the country recognized the need for changes in the health care system and realized that political action was a way to accomplish this change. In 1974, ANA established its PAC — *Nurses' Coalition for Action in Politics (N-CAP)*. In 1985, because of Federal Election Commission (FEC) regulations requiring the coupling of the parent organization's name with the title of each PAC, N-CAP was officially changed to ANA PAC by the ANA House of Delegates governing body.

ANA PAC provides support to candidates for the Senate and House of Representatives and is currently the sixth largest health care PAC in the country. Between 1987 and 1990, ANA PAC had 9,400 contributors with an average donation of $26 per person. In the 1992 election, ANA PAC contributed more than $306,000 to congressional candidates; endorsing 260. Of that number, 192 won election, 62 lost, four retired, and two faced run-off elections. In the 1990 election, $287,000 was contributed by ANA PAC to 243 candidates for federal office. These were both incumbents and challengers, with over 30 percent of the contributions going to the latter. ANA PAC makes special efforts to support challengers sympathetic to its positions – specifically women and people of color — early in their campaigns. Of all the candidates who received ANA PAC support in the 1989-1990 election cycle, 89 percent were elected to office.

GOALS

The goal of the ANA PAC is to improve the health care of the people of this country. It allows nurses to have a collective and powerful voice on issues of fundamental importance to their profession. This is achieved by working through the political process. ANA PAC assists candidates for federal office who believe in and have demonstrated their support for the legislative objectives of ANA. The PAC also educates ANA's members about the political process and candidates' positions on health care and other nursing issues. ANA's political effectiveness stems from the thousands of nurses who contribute money to the PAC, work in political campaigns, and take the time to communicate nursing's positions to their elected officials. In turn, nurses acquire visibility, credibility, and influence.

CONTRIBUTIONS

ANA PAC is made up of the members of ANA who financially support its political positions. The PAC can only solicit funds from a designated group consisting of the parent organization's (ANA's) members, its executives, administrative personnel, and their families. All contributions are voluntary donations. Non-solicited contributions, however, may be accepted from anyone outside the designated group. Funds are collected and placed in a bank account separate from ANA monies. Although association monies support the administrative functioning of the PAC, no ANA funds are used for candidate support.

RELATIONSHIP TO ANA

ANA PAC is housed within the ANA Department of Governmental Affairs. The governing body of ANA PAC is its board of trustees. ANA governmental affairs staff (including the political action director, grassroots coordinator, field representatives, and lobbyists) work very closely with the ANA PAC.

The ANA PAC's function is not limited to soliciting and donating funds for political campaigns. Of even greater importance is its political education function. ANA staff develop workshops and educational materials to enhance the political skills of nurses and make nurses more visible to Members of Congress. They work with ANA's valuable grassroots network (the congressional district coordinator/Senate coordinator network), so that every Member has a politically astute nurse as a contact in his or her state or congressional district.

The staff facilitate fund-raising for ANA PAC and serve as liaison with each SNA, the ANA PAC Board of Trustees, and the candidates in the endorsement process.

ANA's lobbyists also are instrumental in making contact and educating Members on issues of importance to nursing. They attend fund-raisers and task force meetings and work in coalitions with other health care and nursing groups to maximize their impact on those who craft policy at the federal level.

ENDORSEMENT PROCESS

The ANA PAC endorsement process for federal candidates begins at the state level. A representative from the SNA and/or the congressional district coordinator/Senate coordinator must meet with the candidate requesting ANA PAC support to discuss ANA's legislative agenda and the specific concerns of nurses in the district or state. Evaluations are sent to the ANA PAC Board of Trustees which reviews the record of each candidate; considers recommendations from the states and the ANA PAC director; and decides which candidates deserve an ANA PAC endorsement and/or financial contribution. A local group of SNA nurses usually presents the check to the political candidate in the home state.

ENDORSEMENTS

The process of deciding whom to support and formalizing that selection is an involved one. When an organization decides to endorse or support a candidate for political office, it does so for a variety of reasons. The endorsement allows the organization to help its friends — those public officials who, through the course of their careers, have been supportive of its interests. In some races where there may not be a clear indication as to which candidate to support, the endorsement process can open lines of communication between the grassroots lobbyists and the candidate, and lay the groundwork for additional access to the candidate. Endorsement increases the organization's visibility, creating a newsworthy story of a professional group endorsing a candidate for public office.

The PAC's ability to make an endorsement is linked directly to the amount of information available on a particular candidate — how an incumbent has voted, how accessible his or her staff is, and how helpful he or she is on a particular issue. Similarly, although challengers do not have voting records, it is important to have a sense of how they operate and their views on important issues. This requires local input, and, as a result, every organization/association member who is interested in politics should operate constantly as an "intelligence agent" for his or her group. If the information is not available, you should develop specific questions to pose to the candidate. The interview process is invaluable in pinpointing the candidate's positions on specific issues, beyond the campaign rhetoric. Be sure to craft your questions to require more than a "yes" or "no" answer. Remember: information makes the endorsement process work effectively.

The key to making a meaningful endorsement is an open and objective endorsement process. It is essential that the group (within an organization) that is responsible for making the endorsement decision must make public the criteria used and the reasons for each decision. A PAC's mission is not only to endorse a candidate or give financial contributions to the endorsed candidate, but to know that the endorsement is representative of the organization as a whole, not just a few of its members. If individuals feel isolated from the process, if they feel that the decision was not reached in a fair manner, then they will not be influenced by the endorsement and it becomes a hollow gesture.

It also is essential to maintain a sense of perspective about endorsements. Obviously, they are very helpful to your grassroots campaign. However, many once promising politicians — now private citizens — have learned endorsements do not win elections. No one should feel that the task is complete after a candidate has received a PAC endorsement. In fact, the real work has just begun: it is time to get out and actually work for the endorsed candidate.

VOTER REGISTRATION DRIVES

In a political campaign, you need votes to win the election and you can only get those votes from registered voters. A political campaign must build its base first, and, second, develop a source of power.

You may have seen voter registration tables set up at public functions (e.g., country fairs) or in public places (e.g., shopping malls). And, you probably also have seen many volunteers "working the tables," registering people to vote. Organizations and coalitions whose staff volunteer to work voter-registration booths know that increasing the number of registered voters and targeting where registration activities take place can be key components of winning a political election. When your group or coalition decides to conduct a voter registration drive, careful planning is necessary to ensure success.

STEP 1. SETTING UP THE COMMITTEE

Your group should appoint a person to act as coordinator of your voter registration project. This person is responsible for working with registration officials, helping plan the event, and delegating tasks. In addition to the coordinator, a steering committee should be appointed to take on specific tasks and responsibilities such as researching local election laws, recruiting volunteers to conduct the registration drive, promoting publicity in the community, and finding an appropriate place to hold the drive.

STEP 2. RESEARCHING ELECTION LAWS

Every state has different election laws, and many counties have specific registration requirements. It is necessary for you to research these laws before proceeding with the voter registration drive. Contact your state and county elections offices to receive full information.

First, determine the type of registration procedure used in your area (i.e., post card registration, *deputy registration* [i.e., people are certified to register other voters], *centralized registration* [i.e., people must go to a central place, such as a post office, to register] then, obtain additional information to be an informed volunteer:

- What are the address, telephone number, and hours of operation of the local registration office?
- Where does one obtain the necessary registration forms?
- How many days before an election must a voter register?
- What identification is necessary for people to register?
- What are the residency requirements for registration?
- What documentation must a naturalized citizen have to register?
- Is party affiliation required at the time of registration?
- How does a registered voter change his or her party affiliation?
- What registration provisions are made for disabled voters?
- What languages are the registration materials available in?
- May I obtain a copy of the lists of registered voters and/or purged voters from election officials to use during the voter registration drive?

STEP 3. PLANNING YOUR REGISTRATION DRIVE

After you have researched the rules and regulations concerning voter registration drives in your area, develop a calendar of events to help you plan the allotted time for the drive. First and foremost, be sure you have sufficient lead time to register voters before the registration deadline. If there is an active coalition of women's organizations or health care groups in your community, you may wish to join them or set up your own coalition of local groups to work on a joint voter-registration drive. Break down the registration drive into distinct tasks and determine who will accomplish each task and when that task will be done.

The type of registration drive will depend on the local rules. If you reside in a state that allows postcard or deputy registration, you will be able to hold a day or week of registration activities when and where you choose. If you reside in an area that has branch or centralized registration procedures, your options are more limited.

If you live in an area that allows you to register potential voters yourself, you must find a place to hold your drive. Plan to do so in areas that attract large groups of people — shopping malls, grocery stores, workplaces, banks, churches, day care facilities, post offices, and other public places. Be sure to ask permission before you plan to use a site. Provide transportation to potential voters who otherwise could not get to the registration sites.

Next, decide when you will hold your drive. To get adequate numbers of both volunteers and registered voters, keep the time period short (e.g., a Saturday in a shopping mall, one week of lunch hours in the hospital). Schedule your drive around national or community events to spark interest and generate publicity. Some notable periods each year include: Women's History Month (March), Women's Equity Day (August 26), the Fourth of July, and

Mother's Day (May). Build your drive around an activity — e.g., local festivals, picnics, Memorial Day festivities, candidate forums, marches, or sports events.

If you are planning a door-to-door registration drive, organize a walk-a-thon or rally to garner attention and support. Identifying unregistered voters in your community — from lists available from the county elections office — enables you to concentrate your efforts where they will be the most productive. Be sure to work the neighborhood when people are most likely to be at home.

Prior to the actual registration drive, you will want to hold a meeting with your volunteers and train them in registration procedures.

STEP 4. PUBLICIZING YOUR REGISTRATION DRIVE

Prepare and distribute in your community flyers, announcements, and signs on when and where the event will be held. Flyers should be brief, but informative. Emphasize the importance of registering to vote. Ask your hospital, local banks, and grocery stores to post your announcements.

STEP 5. CONDUCTING YOUR REGISTRATION DRIVE

Confirm arrangements with the site of registration, registration officials, and your volunteers prior to the event. During the drive, be courteous and helpful to those registering. Check the registration cards to make sure they are completed properly. If you are using postcards, collect the cards and deliver them to the board of election office in your area. If you live in an area that straddles two counties or states, you may wish to have materials from both areas available.

Keep a list of every person you have registered, so that you may contact them later in your "get-out-the-vote" activities. At the end, thank all of those whose help allowed you to have a successful registration drive.

STEP 6. GET-OUT-THE-VOTE CAMPAIGNS

The registration of voters is useless unless those voters cast a ballot. Studies have shown that if there is no follow-up to voter registration activities, less than 20 percent of those newly registered will go to the polls. A get-out-the-vote campaign on Election Day will help make sure newly registered voters actually go to the polls. If you contact those individuals just prior to Election Day, over 65 percent of them will vote.

The key is providing motivation to potential voters to cast their ballots. As you did with your registration drive, publicize the need to vote through literature, press releases, and public service announcements. This time, the message should emphasize the importance of each individual's vote. In addition, provide information on the date of the election, the location of the polling places, and the hours of operation. Phone canvassing is a useful method to get out the vote. Use the list from your voter registration drive and call the newly registered voters. Congratulate them on their new status and urge them to go to the polls.

Providing services to certain groups of voters also increases turnout. For example, providing day care for those who find it difficult to leave their children at home, or arranging transportation for the elderly or disabled allows people to get to the polls. Often, local bus or taxi companies will help provide transportation for this public service. Giving out information on absentee balloting is a useful service to those who will not be in the area on Election Day. Check with election officials on local requirements for absentee ballots.

A note for federal employees and non-profit organizations: Although federal employees are prohibited by the Hatch Act from engaging in political activities (**See Appendix I**, p. 138) and non-profit organizations are prohibited from doing so by their tax status, a voter registration drive *conducted in a nonpartisan manner* (i.e., no organizational endorsements, political party banners, or literature during the event) is permissible under the law.

COMMUNICATION

An effective political campaign is one that communicates with the voters. Because the standard methods of communication (e.g., mail) often are expensive, there are other political communication techniques you will need to utilize in your campaign.

LITERATURE DISTRIBUTION

Organize volunteers to walk through a neighborhood and drop off literature at every house. This service is invaluable to political candidates who are trying to deliver their message to every voter.

INTRA-ORGANIZATIONAL COMMUNICATION

Communicate with the members in your own organization, network, or coalition by sending out a mailing describing why health care professionals should support a certain candidate. The key to writing effective letters is to keep your audience in mind. The more relevant the message is to the needs, values, and desires of its readers, the more effective it is. Write your letters remembering what you like and dislike about the political mail you receive. Most people appreciate and remember letters that demonstrate a bit of creativity.

TELEPHONE BANKS

Phone banks are invaluable political tools. When you need to communicate in a timely fashion and the message is relatively brief, telephones are the best option. In campaigns, phone banks are used primarily for voter identification programs which call registered voters and determine if they support your candidate or have any specific issues concerns that the candidate can address. If so, you can personalize future communications to the voters.

MAIL

In every political campaign, there is at least one *mass mailing.* To put one together, recruit volunteers who are willing to sit around a table and fold letters, address and stuff envelopes, and lick stamps. If you have a particularly large mailing, you may want to use professional mailing services.

POLITICAL CONTRIBUTIONS

Money is the lifeblood of politics; it propels and wins political campaigns. Because making political contributions or having a well-funded PAC will greatly increase your political clout, you should develop some fund-raising skills.

The best way to get money for a cause is to ask for it. It sounds simpler than it is. Most people are reluctant to ask a good friend to contribute to something they believe in. No one likes to ask friends for money; you know that their budgets are tight and that they probably think they cannot afford to contribute, but the worst thing they can tell you is "no."

There is no point in beating around the bush when asking for a political contribution. The best method is, "Darlene, I am trying to raise money for the Hawaii nurses political action committee. Can you contribute $40 ?"

Start with your personal friends; they probably already know about your involvement with your organization. Next, approach your professional community.

There are several traditional methods of raising money.

FUND-RAISING EVENTS

You can hold an event, inviting people to attend a gathering (e.g., a party, a dinner, a brunch, a reception, or a brown bag lunch) and asking them for contributions. Some people prefer to surprise their guests and ask them for a contribution once they have arrived at the event; others prefer to be upfront and indicate in the invitation that they are hosting a fund-raiser.

It increases attendance and visibility for your fund-raising events if you have *"a draw"* — anything that attracts attention and encourages people to attend. Some organizations use political figures as their "big names." If you do not have a draw, try "a thing." For example, is there a fancy house in your neighborhood where everyone is "just dying to see the kitchen?" Approach the owners to see if they will allow the event to be held there, and let people pay for the privilege of being invited to see this fabulous house.

AUCTIONS

It may be possible to get celebrities you know or who support your cause to contribute some identifiable item for you to auction. For example, a governor might contribute a pen used to sign a significant bill, or a mayor might be willing to take the highest bidder to lunch. Bidding for a popular item can become intense, and, as a result, you can raise a great deal of money relatively easily.

PHONE-A-THONS

Phone-a-thons use the same techniques used in phone banks. Instead of seeking votes, however, you are seeking money. Use your volunteers and a uniform script and call the members in your organization, urging them to make financial pledges. Once you have a verbal promise, follow up and request and collect the money.

DIRECT MAIL

The key to a successful direct-mail effort is to select a proven target audience, then write a letter which focuses on the themes and arguments which you think will move them enough to write out a check. A general mailing to all your members should bring in enough money to cover the costs of the mailing, though it may be relatively advantageous simply to mail a solicitation to people who have contributed previously.

Raising money can be easy or difficult, but it must be legal. If you are raising money for a political campaign, the primary responsibility for knowing and complying with regulations rests with you. Work with individuals who are familiar with the laws and can advise you on your responsibilities. Each state has its own rules and regulations governing political fund-raising. Almost invariably, these are extremely detailed and have a number of requirements.

POLITICAL NETWORKS

A basic truth of politics is that numbers count. Whether the goal is electing someone to office or enacting legislation, politicians have to be able to count votes. Organizations and individuals who want to have political influence have to be able to deliver votes. The best way to help someone deliver those votes is to establish your own base of operation — your own political network.

As a nurse, you are fortunate to have a natural base: one in every 44 registered voters is a nurse. In each congressional district, there are 4,000 to 7,000 nurses. These are impressive numbers. But, there is a vast difference between simply having a base and being able to deliver it, between being able to count a large number of members, and having a large number of members whose votes you can depend on; between people who care about a problem and people who care enough to work for a solution.

If you want to exert some pressure on an elected official or support a candidate, you need people to help you do it. Start with your friends. Use those friends to reach others. Just as you were able to find four or five or six people who are interested in forming a political network, these people, in turn, have four, five, or six others they can recruit to join you.

After you have gathered your initial group, you will want to organize. Your organization does not have to be formal or permanent. Your first task may be simply to grow and develop a method of operation. Establish a system which enables you to communicate quickly and effectively.

You may assign people by workplace — one person/one workplace — a system of communication whereby one person assumes primary responsibility for coordinating and communicating with a group of volunteers in that workplace. In a hospital, for example, you can establish a work site coordinator charged with the overall task of coordinating the work of political volunteers in that hospital. You can assign people by neighborhoods. Give each person the responsibility for coordinating the volunteers and activities in a specific neighborhood.

You will need to know who wants to help and how they can help. You can never have too much information about potential workers. You will need to know their names, work and home addresses and telephone numbers; types of work they would like to do; times they are available; party affiliations; issue interests; past political work; relationships with public officials; list of organizations to which they belong; congressional districts in which they reside; and whether they are registered to vote.

Once you have had a successful campaign or fund-raising drive, you can decide whether you want to make your organization permanent. A permanent network of health care professionals, who are also political veterans, will prove to be a valuable resource as you proceed with your grassroots legislative campaigns. Remember, however, not to work your volunteers too hard. Always be thankful for them: treat them with respect and kindness.

POLITICAL ACTION AND LEGISLATIVE RESULTS

You have gathered your volunteers, you have held a voter registration drive, you have raised money for a political campaign, you have volunteered at the phone bank, and you have gone door to door getting the votes out on Election Day. Your candidate has won. A job well done — he or she could not have been elected without your help and the help of your volunteers. Is your work finished?

Not yet. The reason you participated in all these activities was to elect a candidate who represented your views. Now it is time to let your views be known. If your candidate was elected to Congress, before he or she travels to Washington, DC, call and arrange a meeting with that newly elected Member in your home district. The most effective time to lobby a public official is when his or her memories of your help in the campaign are fresh. Develop a one-page fact sheet describing three to four specific issue areas of concern. Explain what you would like to see that person accomplish in his or her first term.

By arranging this first meeting, you have established yourself as a grassroots lobbyist and opened the lines of communication on legislative issues with your new Member of Congress.

FOR FURTHER INFORMATION

For further information on the ANA PAC, fund-raising, and organizing a campaign, contact the:

ANA PAC Director
Department of Governmental Affairs
American Nurses Association
600 Maryland Avenue, SW
Suite 100 West
Washington, DC 20024-2571
Telephone: (202) 554-4444

THE MEDIA*

Half the battle in a grassroots lobbying campaign is fought in the public arena. Educating the public on the need for health care reform will prompt people to voice their views on the subject, acting as catalysts for congressional action. An essential agent in this public education is the media. Using the press to publicize your issue will provide you with a free advertisement, getting your message to more people than your volunteer coalition could ever begin to contact.

When you prepare a news release, you must tell the reader or listener the basics: who, what, when, where, why, and how. Information conveyed through the media must be newsworthy. News is what people need to know. If you tell people what they need to know and why they need to know it, they will pay attention.

To be newsworthy, your information must have at least one of the following characteristics:

- Timeliness. It is current, or possesses an angle or slant that makes it seem new.
- Proximity. It has immediate impact on the audience's geographic area.
- Magnitude. It involves a considerable number of people or amount of money, for example.
- Star Appeal. It has to do with a local or national celebrity.
- Human Interest. It has a personal appeal and offers drama, conflict, or the unusual.
- Impact. It affects the audience's daily lives, and can be related effectively from the audience's perspective.

DEVELOPING YOUR PRESS LIST

Your goal is to get basic information to reporters and producers. To start your media campaign (which should be an integral part of your grassroots lobbying campaign), develop a press list. Begin by scanning television guides, local newspapers, and radio programs. Call the television and radio stations (listed in the local yellow pages) and ask for the names of the producer and the news and public service directors. Add the names of any television reporters who have covered relevant issues in the past. List all daily and

---

* This Chapter was adapted from: *Public Information Manual,* 1990. Kansas City, Mo: American Nurses Association.

weekly newspapers published in your area. Call each newspaper and obtain the names of the city editor, the business editor, and the editorial page editor. Find out who regularly covers health issues.

If you are in a large city, check to see if there is an Associated Press (AP) or United Press International (UPI) regional bureau in your area. In addition, check whether *Newsweek, Time,* the *New York Times,* or other large newspapers or magazines have local bureaus. If so, add the names of the bureau chiefs to your list. Update your list on a regular basis.

An accurate, up-to-date media list is almost as important as the news you are promoting. Your news release or news conference or other publicity must get to the right editor or reporter to be broadcast or published. Sending your information to the wrong person or the wrong station will waste both time and money. A lifestyle editor probably will not use a news release about direct reimbursement legislation.

TYPES OF PRESS VEHICLES

Different types of media exist for different purposes. Tailoring your story to fit the needs of a specific media vehicle will greatly increase your chances of getting your story covered.

GENERAL INTEREST NEWSPAPERS

- Concentrate more on informing than other media, and less on entertaining.
- Can accommodate complex information.
- Reach a broad socio-economic audience.
- Range in coverage from news to special interest features.
- Contact person varies with size and frequency of publication:
  - small weeklies: editor.
  - large weeklies and semi-weeklies: editor, managing editor, or news editor.
  - medium to large dailies: department editor, city editor, news editor.

MAGAZINES

- Pinpoint specific audiences.
- Provide investigative/interpretive reporting and in-depth analysis of complex issues.
- Maintain permanent records.
- Offer access to important audiences.
- Contact person: managing editor, department editor.
- Contact time: minimum two months lead time.

WIRE SERVICES

- Ensure immediate and widespread coverage.
- Usually increase other media's acceptance of information.
- Economical vehicles for disseminating information.
- Contact person: local or regional bureau chief.

FIGURE 20

RULES FOR WORKING WITH PRINT MEDIA

→ Give news first, then explain background.
→ Use dramatic statistics and facts.
→ Speak in outlines.
→ Speak slowly and concisely.

PR WIRES

- Electronic distribution of news releases to media.
- Offer feature and specialized news services.
- Originator of information pays a fee.
- Contact: sales representatives.

RADIO

- Mobile medium which reaches drive-time audience.
- Offers formats that draw specific audiences.
- Hourly or regularly scheduled newscasts.
- FM stations reach a larger audience than AM stations.
- Contact: News directors, producers.

TELEVISION

- Attracts the average American's attention for 27 hours a week.
- Serves as primary news source for 65 percent of all Americans.
- Essentially an entertainment medium.
- Contact: Assignment editor, program director.

CABLE TELEVISION

- Reaches 50 percent of all households with television.
- Offers local channels for special interest/public affairs.
- Contact: program director.

FIGURE 21

RULES FOR WORKING WITH ELECTRONIC MEDIA

→ Speak in twenty-second sentences ("sound bites").
→ Speak in short sentences.
→ Include the question in your answer.
→ Don't talk "above" the audience.
→ Use visual aids (if television).
→ Don't ramble.
→ Be concise.
→ Use analogies.

THE NEWS RELEASE

Your primary contact with the media will be through a *news (or press) release*. Whether you are advising the media of a press conference, issuing a statement, or providing background material, your news release will be the single most important document in attracting the media's attention. A sample press release is provided in Figure 22.

FIGURE 22

SAMPLE
PRESS
RELEASE

NEWS RELEASE

American Nurses Association
600 Maryland Avenue SW
Suite 100 West
Washington, DC 20024-2571
TEL 202 554 4444
FAX 202 554 2262

FOR IMMEDIATE RELEASE   CONTACT: Joan Meehan, ext. 244
January 22, 1993   202/554-4444

**AMERICAN NURSES ASSOCIATION PRAISES CLINTON FOR "REMOVING GAG"
ON NURSES WHO PROVIDE COUNSELING IN FAMILY PLANNING CLINICS**

WASHINGTON, DC – The American Nurses Association (ANA) praised President Clinton, who today rescinded the so-called "gag rule" by executive order, thus allowing women to receive full counseling about reproductive health choices in federally funded family planning clinics.

ANA President Virginia Trotter Betts, JD, MSN, RN, who was at the White House for the signing of the order, said, "Nursing's fundamental belief is that all patients must have full and accurate information in order to make informed choices about their care. We are here today to thank President Clinton for allowing nurses to fulfill our ethical and professional responsibility to our women patients."

Nurse practitioners and nurse midwives are the bulk of professional and licensed staff within the nation's 4,000 family planning clinics. Early last year, the Bush Administration reversed the "gag rule" for physicians, but retained it for nurses and other nonphysician providers.

"This action demonstrates President Clinton's commitment to increase access to care and his understanding that nurses are qualified to provide essential front-line health care," Betts said. "It is a victory for both patients and nurses to know that health care professionals' right to free speech will not be restrained under a Clinton Administration."

The American Nurses Association is the only full-service professional organization representing the nation's 2 million Registered Nurses through its 53 constituent associations. ANA advances the nursing profession by fostering high standards of nursing practice, promoting the economic and general welfare of nurses in the workplace, projecting a positive and realistic view of nursing, and by lobbying the Congress and regulatory agencies on health care issues affecting nurses and the public.

###

The news release should disseminate information efficiently. It will be judged on the basis of its interest to an audience or target medium, its timeliness, and its adaptability to use by the media vehicle. It should be printed on 8-1/2" x 11" paper with the name of your organization or coalition, date of issue, and a contact person clearly identified. The news release should never exceed two double-spaced typed pages.

In the top left corner of the first page, type FOR IMMEDIATE RELEASE or RELEASE ON RECEIPT to indicate the time intended for the release of information contained in the news release. If the release is to be held (*embargoed*), indicate the time of release. Remember the news media have no legal responsibility to honor this embargo, though they usually will. In the top right corner, print the name of the organization's contact person and telephone number. This person will be called by any interested media.

Move down the first page, about one inch, and type the headline. It should be catchy and entice the reader to continue reading the release. After the headline, type the body of the release. Do not split paragraphs between pages. If the copy exceeds one page, type "-more-" at the bottom center of each page, except the last. Indicate the end of the text by typing "30" or "#" at the bottom center.

The lead sentence of your news release should answer the primary questions about the story. Make your points clearly. Follow the "inverted pyramid" style of writing in which the importance of your information diminishes as you progress through the story. Be sure the content, spelling, grammar, and punctuation are accurate and correct.

Use short, simple sentences with subject and verb in clear relationship. Average twenty words per sentence. Follow unusual names with phonetic spellings in parentheses. Read the copy aloud when you are finished to evaluate it for quality and content.

MEDIA ADVISORIES

A *media advisory* is designed to alert the media about upcoming events (e.g., press conferences) and generate on-the-scene coverage. In this type of news release, you provide enough information to entice reporters to cover your event to get the story. Give a brief listing of the facts, such as a description of the event along with its scheduled time and place, and identify opportunities for interviews. Distribute a media advisory approximately two weeks in advance of the event, if possible, to allow editors time to schedule coverage.

LEAD OR TIP SHEETS

A *lead or tip sheet* is designed to generate media interest in local issues. It usually runs one page and has three to five capsulized descriptions regarding an issue's local impact. This is intended to produce feature stories, not hard news coverage. It is very useful in generating broad, general interest in your legislative issues.

FACT SHEETS

Fact sheets provide statistics, definitions, and background on a particular legislative subject. Because the media uses fact sheets as references to answer frequently asked questions, fact sheets containing detailed data can be very useful. For example, illustrations and data on health care costs in your community could be used by both public officials and journalists.

BACKGROUNDERS

A *backgrounder* provides basic information on specific issues. This information should be sent to the media prior to an interview or news conference or utilized as a reference document. The backgrounder should be from one to two pages long. By providing the reporter with some background information in advance, face-to-face interviews can be more thorough.

THE OP-ED PIECE

An *op-ed* column is written in editorial form and analyzes an issue or event from the perspective of an individual or organization. A newspaper's op-ed page usually appears on the page opposite the editorial page. It can play an important role in your lobbying strategy.

Op-Ed columns are signed by "guest editors" (i.e., people recognized as experts in their respective fields) and submitted to newspapers for publication. They allow the newspaper's readers to present an opinion in more depth than is possible with a letter to the editor. By studying the style of previously published op-eds, you get a clue to the format and approach most likely to appeal to the editor who selects op-eds.

A typical op-ed should be 600 to 800 words long. Write a strong first paragraph that grabs the reader's attention. Use short paragraphs, not exceeding three or four sentences each. State your opinions in the op-ed piece and do not quote other people. Be certain that the op-ed stands by itself; do not assume the reader has any prior knowledge about the issue. Do not use acronyms, abbreviations, or jargon. Make certain that a reader unfamiliar with your subject will be able to understand the op-ed.

Op-ed submissions should be sent to the editorial page editor or, with small newspapers, to the publisher. Provide a background sentence about the author, including his or her affiliation and whatever else qualifies him or her as an expert on the subject.

An extremely effective approach is to write one op-ed piece and distribute it to contacts, in your state, who have some name recognition. For example, an op-ed on the subject of maternal and child health funding could be sent to the president of the state's nurses association, the state education association, the state Gray Panther's organization, and a prominent member of the state legislature. Select people who agree with your position, but might not have time to write an article themselves. Ask each of these people (hopefully, in different parts of the state) to approach the editors of their local papers and submit the op-ed under their name. It will seem as if a number of prestigious organizations and people are writing opinion pieces on maternal and child health issues, thus focusing increased attention on the issue.

THE PRESS CONFERENCE

Call a press conference *only if you have something very important to say*. There is nothing more depressing than holding a press conference that no one attends. Send out a media advisory telling the press why you are holding the press conference. Do not give them enough information to write a story without attending.

Remember, the human interest angle is very important. What effects does your proposal have on people's lives? One example is the very effective press conference — held on the issue of family and medical leave several years ago — which consisted of families from around the country getting up one by one and telling their stories of losing their jobs when they had to stay home and care for a newborn child or sick relative.

Do not hold a press conference when:

- the information you are generating is only of interest to a small segment of the media;
- a news release, or other written form of individual contact will suffice;
- you or the organization you represent is unprepared to answer questions beyond the content of your prepared statement.

If you have decided that your announcement warrants a press conference, determine the specific goals for the conference, including what content areas are to be covered. Schedule the conference to accommodate local media requirements:

- 9:30 a.m. to 10:00 a.m. for that evening's newspapers.
- no later than 2:00 p.m. for the next morning's newspapers and evening television newscasts.

Send your media advisory seven days in advance of the press conference and follow up with personal telephone calls to individual journalists. List yourself on the local *daybook* listing of events, produced by the wire services. Include a fact sheet outlining the general subject of the press conference, the spokesperson's name, and the time and place of the conference. Prepare supporting materials such as news releases, opening statements, backgrounders, and fact sheets for *press kits*.

Draft possible questions and your responses. Hold a mock news conference with the spokesperson before the actual event. You cannot be too prepared.

Immediately before the start of the press conference, make sure you have completed all the tasks listed in Figure 23, **"Press Conference Checklist,"** p 108.

FIGURE 23

PRESS CONFERENCE CHECKLIST

❏ Press kits are available at entrance to press conference.
❏ Microphones have been tested.
❏ Seating is arranged in such a manner that reporters can see and hear clearly.
❏ Head table with podium is present.
❏ Space has been left between head table and audience for photographers.
❏ Room is brightly lit.
❏ Writing materials have been provided.
❏ Electrical outlets have been checked.
❏ Tape recorder is set up.
❏ Sign-in book for media representatives is at entrance to press conference.

Designate a person to welcome each journalist and be available to answer questions regarding the format of the press conference and identity of the spokesperson(s). The opening statement should be no longer than two to three minutes. Distribute a written statement if what you have to say takes up more time. No one person should speak for more than five minutes and no more than three people should speak.

After the statements have been completed, the person who made the opening statement should field questions from the journalists. When the questions begin to wane, the convener announces that time is limited and just two additional questions will be heard. After the final questions, the convener closes the press conference and thanks the media for coming.

After the press conference, be sure to follow up as necessary. Comply quickly with any requests for individual interviews and additional information, but do not deviate from the primary content of the news conference. Remember that no conversation is off the record. Be sure that all reporters have all the information and visuals they need. Schedule some time after the press conference for debriefing. Replay and critique the recorded interview.

Make arrangements to monitor print and broadcast coverage after the press conference to determine what impact your press conference had.

THE LETTER TO THE EDITOR

Writing a *letter to the editor* is an easy way to publicize your own opinions and to reach a large segment of the population at no cost. But, there is no way to ensure that your letter will be included in the "Letters to the Editor" section of the newspaper. Your chances will increase if you sign your letter as the head of a coalition or organization.

THE RADIO INTERVIEW

Radio interviews are another means of publicizing your ideas. If you agree to a request to be on the radio — either as part of a news broadcast or a radio interview show — listen to that particular program several times before your scheduled appearance to familiarize yourself with the format, the host, the style, the tempo, and the types of callers (if it is a call-in show). Prepare five key points on your subject and practice making them, using short, crisp, quick sentences. Write out possible questions you may be asked and plan short answers. Do not use complicated statistics, acronyms, technical terminology, or jargon. Assume that the audience has no prior knowledge of the subject matter. Develop a local angle on your issue so that it is relevant to the city or state where the program airs. Anticipate hostile questions and practice answering them in a clear and forceful manner.

When answering the interviewer's questions, place the most important points at the beginning of each of your responses. Always refer to the interviewer by name, but do not overdo it. Be energetic, involved, and direct.

If the interviewer asks a complex question, do not respond instantly; pause briefly and organize your response. Answer those parts of the question with which you feel most comfortable. Although your mind may be racing ahead in anticipation, speak slowly when answering.

Never lie during an interview. Do not be afraid to admit you do not know. Promise to find the answer and follow up with the interviewer.

Finally, until you have left the studio, do not say anything you do not want to hear broadcast. *Nothing is off the record.*

THE TELEVISION INTERVIEW

The television interview is not much different in substance from the radio interview. The difference is that the audience can see you. If possible, view the television program you have been invited to appear on before your scheduled visit. Become familiar with the color of the backdrop and types of furniture used, and dress according to the set. Wear business-type clothing — e.g., a suit and a blouse with no bows or ties at the neck (for women), and a traditional suit (for men). Wear solid colors, and avoid colors that tend to blend in with your skin as well as fabrics with a high sheen.

It is true that the television camera adds ten pounds. Wear slightly more make-up than usual, but not so much as to give yourself a clown-like appearance. Make sure that your hair is neat-looking and style it so that it will not fall in your face during the interview. Avoid a lot of jewelry, scarves, and other accessories.

When you are on camera, pay attention to your posture. You will not be taken seriously if you are slumping. Use hand gestures to help you appear animated, but contain them so that your arms do not fly out of the picture. Discuss broad issues instead of focusing on technicalities. Whenever possible, make your remarks relevant to the locale. Be very careful not to drone on in front of a television camera. Speak in short sentences.

Use your host's name and engage him or her in conversation as much as possible. Discussions are always more interesting than monologues. If you are going to give an address to which viewers can write for information or materials, advise the producer of the television show in advance so that it can be superimposed on the screen during the interview. Then you do not have to repeat it.

FIGURE 24

MEDIA INTERVIEW CHECKLIST

❏ **Practice, practice, practice before an interview.**
❏ **Research the media outlet.**
❏ **Anticipate questions.**
❏ **Speak in short sentences.**
❏ **Discuss broad issues, avoid technicalities.**
❏ **Everything you say is "on the record."**
❏ **Don't bluff – Don't be afraid to say you don't know.**

THE PAID ADVERTISEMENT

A number of national associations recently have used paid advertisements to get their messages out. Organizations have taken full-page ads in the *New York Times* and the *Washington Post* to further their causes. This method garners a lot of attention, but the cost is prohibitive. A full-page ad in the *Washington Post* currently costs approximately $35,000.

HOW TO HANDLE THE PRESS: STRATEGIES

There are tremendous opportunities to reach the public through the media. If your media outreach efforts are well-organized and well-planned, they will be successful.

BE SENSITIVE TO DEADLINES

Reporters work under tremendous deadline pressure. Often, a reporter is assigned to several stories in a single workday and only has a short time in which to gather information, find interviewees, conduct interviews, and file a story. As the source, the easier you make the reporter's job, the more likely it is that the information you offer will make it into print or on the air.

ASK DEADLINES

When a reporter calls, ask if he or she is on a deadline and when the information is needed. Sometimes, a reporter is calling to get preliminary background information; at other times, he or she is looking for quotes to finalize a story. Be sure to clarify what the reporter is seeking and tailor your answer accordingly.

KEEP REGULAR CONTACTS WITH THE MEDIA

Most reporters and editors cover many different issues. Regular contacts with the media are absolutely essential to effective media work. The best efforts involve contacts with the press from three to six times per year.

USE HUMAN INTEREST ANGLES

The human interest elements of issues help to make the issues understandable to the general public. To maximize the impact your issue has, find people whose situation will drive home its importance.

PIGGYBACK ON OTHER NATIONAL ISSUES

If you know that a congressional hearing is being held on health care reform, or that the Supreme Court is about to hand down a decision on civil rights, or that the Department of Health and Human Services is releasing a report on immunizations, hold a press conference on the national story using your local angle. You can increase the chances of having both the national story and the local story run by your newspapers and television stations.

DO NOT OVERSELL

Use the most appropriate strategy for the news you are releasing. If you have just barely enough information for a press conference, do not hold a press conference. If you should be issuing a statement within hours, do not wait for two days to gather the information you need to write a news release.

GET INFORMATION FROM THE REPORTER

When a reporter calls you, obtain the reporter's name, his or her producer's name, their affiliation, and subject areas they cover as soon as you start the conversation. Add this information to your media file.

ALWAYS FOLLOW UP

When you conclude a conversation with a reporter, ask if he or she has all the information needed, when the story will run, and if you can receive a clip (if it is written). Offer to be available if they need additional information. Make sure all relevant parties are sent any information you promise them.

ADDITIONAL RESOURCES FOR YOUR LOBBYING CAMPAIGN

The ANA produces several publications that can assist you in your grassroots lobbying efforts.

Capital Update, the biweekly legislative and regulatory newsletter of the Department of Governmental Affairs, tells you how *you* can influence congressional and agency decisions (see promotional announcement at back of this book).

Legislative and Regulatory Initiatives is published every two years at the beginning of a new Congress and contains ANA's positions and background statements on issues with an impact on nursing — including nursing education and research programs, Medicare, Medicaid, reimbursement, health care reform, and pension reform.

The American Nurses Association *Congressional Directory,* designed specifically for the ANA, lists all Members of Congress and congressional committees for the current congress.

Grassroots Lobbying: A Great Tool for Nurses is a ten-minute video which contains a wealth of information on basic and advanced grassroots-lobbying techniques, and uses SNA members and their experiences to illustrate how to lobby effectively.

Nurses and Politics: Shaping the Future, a video, shows nurses how to get involved with a political campaign — how to hold fund-raisers, help candidates for political office, and generate community support for political action.

American Nurses Association Congressional District and Senate Coordinator (CDC/SC) Handbook tells you everything you need to know about starting a political and legislative network. It provides ANA congressional district and senate coordinators step-by-step instructions on participating in the political process.

Network News is a newsletter for the ANA Congressional District and Senate Coordinators providing updates on "hot" political and legislative news. Contact the CDC/SC Coordinator in the ANA Department of Governmental Affairs for more information.

For information and order forms for these publications, please contact the Governmental Affairs Department, ANA. Call the Marketing Department for information on and forms for Legislative and Regulatory Initiatives *and the* Congressional Directory.

GLOSSARY OF LEGISLATIVE AND REGULATORY TERMS

Act
The term for legislation that has been passed by both houses of Congress and signed by the president (or passed by Congress in an override of a presidential veto [see *override*]), thus becoming law.

Adjournment Sine Die
Adjournment without definitely fixing a day for reconvening; literally "adjournment without a day." Marks the official end of a congressional session.

Adjournment to a Day Certain
Adjournment under a motion or resolution which fixes the next time of meeting. Neither house can adjourn for more than three days without the concurrence of the other. A session of Congress is not ended by adjournment to a day certain.

Administrative Assistant (AA)
The top aide in a congressional office; often referred to as chief of staff. Duties often can be political as well as administrative.

Amendment
Proposal of a representative or senator to alter the language or provisions in a bill or in another amendment. An amendment usually is debated and voted on in the same manner as a bill.

Amendment in the Nature of a Substitute
An amendment that seeks to replace the entire text of a bill or a large portion of it.

Appropriations Bill
Grants the actual monies authorized by the corresponding authorization bill(s), but not necessarily the total amount specified under the authorization bill. An appropriations bill originates in the House and normally is not acted upon until its authorization measure is enacted. Generally, it cannot provide more money than has been authorized for a particular program under the authorizing legislation.

Authorization Bill
Substantive legislation that establishes or continues the legal operation of a federal program or agency — and its authorized funding levels — either indefinitely or for a specific period of time. An authorization bill usually is a prerequisite for an appropriations bill and sets a ceiling for it.

Bill
Most legislative proposals before Congress are in the form of bills. They are designated as H.R. (House of Representatives) or S. (Senate), according to the chamber in which they originate, and by a number assigned in the order in which they were introduced, starting at the beginning of each two-year Congress. *Public bills* deal with most legislative proposals and become *Public Laws* when approved by Congress and signed by the president. *Private bills* deal with indi-

vidual matters such as claims against the government, immigration and naturalization cases, and land titles, and become *Private Laws* when approved and signed.

"Boll Weevils" — A group of conservative southern Democrat House Members who frequently vote with Republicans on budget and defense issues.

Budget — The document sent to Congress by the president in February of each year. It estimates government revenues and expenditures for the following fiscal year and recommends specific appropriations.

Budget Authority — Authority to enter into obligations which will result in immediate or future payment of federal funds.

Budget Deficit — The amount by which government budget outlays exceed budget receipts for a given fiscal year.

Budget Reconciliation — A procedure to bring tax and spending bills into conformity with levels set in the congressional budget resolutions.

Budget Resolution — A concurrent resolution passed by both houses of Congress — but not requiring the signature of the president — setting forth or revising the congressional version of the federal budget (see *Concurrent Resolution*).

By Request — A phrase used when a Member introduces a bill at the request of an executive agency, but does not necessarily endorse it.

Calendar — An agenda of business awaiting possible action by the chamber. The House uses five legislative calendars — the *Consent, Discharge, House, Private,* and *Union Calendars* — depending on the type of bill. The Senate uses only one legislative calendar, and one non-legislative *(executive)* calendar that is used to schedule debate and votes on treaties and nominations.

Caucus — A group of Members with a common interest. The most powerful are the Democratic and Republican caucuses or conferences in each chamber. There are at least 100 other caucuses representing interests from sugar growers to mushroom growers to shoe producers. Among the larger caucuses are the Congressional Black Caucus and the Congressional Caucus for Women's Issues.

Chairman's Mark — The draft of a bill that the chairman/chairwoman of a committee or subcommittee uses as the starting point in a mark-up.

Chamber — Meeting place for the total membership of either the House or the Senate, as distinguished from offices and committee rooms.

"Christmas Tree" — A legislative measure generously ornamented with unrelated amendments benefiting a wide range of interests. This term is more applicable to Senate than to House bills because of House rules which, unlike those of the Senate, require that amendments be *germane* to the bill.

Clean Bill — Frequently, after a committee has finished a major revision of a bill, one of the committee Members — usually the chairman/chairwoman — will assemble the changes, plus what is left of the original bill, into a new measure and introduce it as a *clean bill* with a new number.

Clerk of the House	Chief administrative officer of the House of Representatives with duties corresponding to those of the Secretary of the Senate.
Cloakroom	The area just off the House and Senate floors where Members can discuss legislation and conduct business in a relaxed atmosphere. Each party in each chamber has its own cloakroom. Outside telephone inquiries can be made to these cloakrooms to find out what business is before the chamber, how a vote came out, who is speaking, and so on.
Cloture	The process whereby debate in the Senate is limited. To be introduced, a cloture motion requires the signatures of 16 senators, and 60 senators (three-fifths of the membership) must vote for cloture in order for it to be invoked. Once cloture is invoked, each senator is limited to one hour of debate.
Closed Rule	The means to prohibit floor introduction of amendments not approved by the committee which brought the bill to the House floor. Under a closed rule, if granted by the Rules Committee at the request of the sponsoring committee, the House must either accept or reject the bill as recommended by that committee. Closed rules usually are limited to tax and Social Security bills which are complicated and highly technical. With other types of legislation, the Rules Committee generally grants some type of *open rule* so that amendments can be considered.
Colloquy	An exchange between two or more Members on the floor during debate on a bill. A colloquy usually is prepared in advance and is designed to give a more detailed explanation of certain provisions of a bill.
Committee	A subdivision of the House or Senate which prepares legislation for action by the parent chamber or conducts investigations as directed. Most standing committees are divided into subcommittees, which study legislation, hold hearings, write legislation, and report their recommendations to the full committee. Only the full committee can report legislation to the full House or Senate for action.
Committee of the Whole	The working title of what is formally *The Committee of the Whole House on the State of the Union.* Unlike other committees, it has no fixed membership, but is comprised of any 100 or more House Members who participate in legislative debate on the floor of the House. Because the Committee of the Whole need number only 100 representatives (instead of the 218 normally required for a quorum), a minimum number required to be present is more readily attained and, therefore, business is expedited. Most noncontroversial bills considered by the House of Representatives are handled in the Committee of the Whole.
Concurrent Resolution	A resolution that must pass both the House and Senate, but does not require the president's signature and does not have the force of law. It is designated as H. Con. Res. or S. Con. Res, depending on the chamber of origin. Concurrent resolutions generally are used to make or amend rules applicable to both houses or to express the

sentiment of the two houses. For example, a concurrent resolution is used to fix the time for adjournment of a Congress. It might also be used to convey the congratulations of Congress to another country on the anniversary of its independence. It serves as the vehicle for coordinated decisions on the federal budget — including the budget resolution — under the 1974 Congressional Budget and Impoundment Control Act (see *Budget Resolution*).

Conference	The meeting between selected members of the House and Senate to iron out the differences between the house-passed and Senate-passed provisions of a bill. The final agreement is called a conference report. It must be approved by both the House and Senate. Members of the conference committee are appointed formally by the Speaker of the House and the presiding officer of the Senate and are called *managers* for their respective chambers.
Congressional Record	The daily printed account of the proceedings in both the House and Senate chambers. Members are allowed to revise their spoken words before they are printed.
Congressional Research Service (CRS)	An arm of the Library of Congress that provides virtually any kind of information or research requested by a Member or congressional staff. The one thing that CRS will not provide is information on another Member's voting record.
Congressional Terms of Office	Begin on January 3 of the year following the general election (odd-numbered years) and ending two years later.
Continuing Resolution	A joint resolution passed by Congress and signed by the president that allows federal agencies to continue to operate at current fiscal-year funding levels until their regular appropriations bills for the next fiscal year are enacted. (Also called *"CR"* or *continuing appropriations*) (see *Joint Resolution*).
Cable-Satellite Public Affairs Network (C-SPAN)	Provides live, gavel-to-gavel television coverage of House and Senate proceedings.
Dear Colleague	A letter from one Member to another (or to all Members of one or both chambers), asking for support for a bill or amendment, or cosponsorship of a particular piece of legislation.
Discharge Petition	In the House, a motion to get a bill out of committee and on to the House floor when the committee refuses to act on the bill. The motion, or petition, requires the signatures of a majority (218 Members) of the House.
District Office	In addition to their Capitol Hill offices, Members usually maintain one or more offices in their congressional districts.
District Work Period	A congressional euphemism for *recess*.
Enacting Clause	Key phrase in bills that states, "Be it enacted by the House of Representatives and Senate..." If passed, a motion to strike it from legislation kills the bill.

Engrossed Bill	The final copy of a bill that has passed the House or the Senate. The text, amended by floor action, is incorporated into the bill. The result, printed on blue paper, is the engrossed bill, which at this point becomes known as an *act,* signifying that it has passed one house of Congress. This engrossed copy is then delivered to the other chamber.
Enrolled Bill	The final copy of a bill that has been passed in identical form by the House and Senate. It is certified to by an officer of the house of origin (clerk of the House or secretary of the Senate) and then sent on for the signatures of the House Speaker, the Senate president, and the president. An enrolled bill is printed on parchment.
Entitlement Program	A federal program — such as Social Security, Medicare, Medicaid, veterans' compensation , or unemployment compensation — that guarantees a certain level of benefits to persons who meet requirements set by law.
Executive Session	Meeting of a committee (or, occasionally, of the entire House or Senate) that is closed to the public and the press (e.g., to discuss national security issues or to mark up tax bills).
Expenditures	The actual spending of funds as distinguished from their appropriation. As required by the Constitution, funds are expended (or spent) by the executive branch. They are appropriated by Congress.
Filibuster	In the Senate, a time-delaying strategy of debate, amendments, other procedures, and just plain talk, used by those in the minority to defeat a proposal favored by the majority or to achieve a compromise on it. The most common filibuster method is to take advantage of the Senate's rules permitting unlimited debate. A filibuster can be stopped only by invoking cloture which requires a 60-senator vote (see *Cloture*).
Fiscal Year	Financial operations of the government are conducted in a twelve-month fiscal year, beginning October l and ending September 30. The fiscal year carries the same number as the calendar year in which it ends.
Five-Minute Rule	A debate-limiting rule of the House, which specifies that while the House is meeting in the Committee of the Whole, a Member offering an amendment may speak for five minutes in its favor, followed by an opponent who also speaks for five minutes.
Floor Manager	The Members who have the task of steering legislation through floor debate and the amendment process to a final vote in the chamber. The floor managers are usually the chairman/chairwoman and ranking minority Member of the committee that reported the legislation to the House or Senate floor.
Frank	A Member's facsimile signature on envelopes, used in lieu of stamps for official outgoing mail, making it postage-free. Also, the privilege of sending mail postage-free.

Germane	Pertaining to the subject of the bill under consideration. All House amendments must be germane. The Senate requires that amendments be germane only when they are proposed to general appropriations bills, bills being considered under cloture, or, often, when proceeding under an agreement to limit debate. The 1974 Budget Act also requires that amendments to concurrent budget resolutions be germane.
Hearings	Committee sessions for hearing witnesses. At hearings on legislation, witnesses generally include specialists, government officials, and spokespersons for individuals and groups considered well-versed in the issues or bills under study.
Hopper	A wooden box on the House clerk's desk where bills are deposited upon introduction. In the Senate, a Member rises at his desk and announces that he or she is introducing a bill. After briefly describing it, the senator hands it to a page who delivers it to a desk in front of the Senate president's rostrum.
House	The House of Representatives, as distinct from the Senate, although each body is termed a *house* of Congress.
House Calendar	Listing of public bills — for action by the House of Representatives — that do not directly or indirectly appropriate money or raise revenue.
Joint Committee	A committee, composed of a specified number of representatives and senators, that studies and reports on specific policy areas (e.g., the Joint Committee on Taxation). A joint committee has no legislative authority.
Joint Resolution	A resolution (designated as H. J. Res. or S. J. Res.) that must pass both the House and Senate and receive the president's signature, just as a bill does. If approved, it has the force of law. Differing in no substantive way from a bill, a joint resolution often is used to address a very limited matter. Joint resolutions are used to propose amendments to the Constitution. They do not require presidential signature and become part of the Constitution when three-fourths of the states have ratified them.
Law	An act of Congress which has been signed by the president, or passed over his or her veto by a two-thirds vote in both houses of Congress.
Legislative Assistant (LA)	A Member's aide who is responsible for legislative duties.
Lame Duck Session	A session of Congress that occurs after the November elections, but before the newly elected Members of the new Congress have been sworn in on January 3.
Line-Item Veto	The authority to veto part, rather than all, of an appropriations bill. The phrase, *line item,* refers to individual accounts within a program or agency that could be vetoed without jeopardizing the entire appropriations bill. Because the president currently does not have line-item veto authority, he or she must veto an entire appropriations bill in order to "veto" funding for a specific account. A number of governors do have line-item veto authority.

Majority Leader	Chief strategist and floor leader for the party in control of the House and/or Senate; elected by Members of the majority party.
Majority Whip	The assistant to the majority leader in both the House and Senate. This person keeps Members advised as to the legislative program, rounds them up for important votes, and keeps his or her party's leadership informed, via *nose counts,* of how many votes they can expect for and against a measure, and from whom.
Mark up	To work on legislation in committee or subcommittee; approving, amending or rejecting each provision and the bill as a whole. If the bill is extensively revised, the new version may be introduced, usually by the committee or subcommittee chairman/chairwoman, as a separate bill with a new number (see *Clean Bill*).
Minority Leader	Floor leader for the minority party in both the House and Senate.
Minority Whip	Chief assistant to the minority leader.
Morning Business	In the Senate, the period at the beginning of each legislative day during which senators may introduce bills or resolutions. Senators also may make speeches on any subject during this time.
Nominations	Appointments, by the president, to executive branch, federal judicial, and diplomatic posts, all subject to Senate confirmation.
Omnibus Bill	A bill containing several separate, but related, legislative proposals.
One-Minutes	Short speeches by House Members at the beginning of each legislative day. The speeches may cover any subject, but are limited to one minute.
Ordered Reported	A full committee approves a bill and *orders it reported* (referred) to the House or Senate. This means that the bill has cleared the committee, but is not quite ready for floor action. First, the committee must write a report explaining the bill and its actions on it. The main body of the report contains the majority views, with minority views and individual views or additional views appended. The bill and report are filed in the House or Senate and at that point, the bill is considered *reported*.
Outlays	Payments made to liquidate obligations incurred by federal agencies or programs (see *Budget Authority)*.
Override	A process whereby Congress rejects, (or overrides), a presidential veto of a bill. It requires a two-thirds vote of the entire membership in each chamber.
Pair	An agreement between Members on opposite sides of an issue whereby a Member who is present during the vote withholds his or her vote so that the absence of the other Member will not affect the outcome of the vote. The names of lawmakers pairing on a given vote and their stands, if known, are printed in the vote tally appearing in the *Congressional Record*. Pairs are not counted in determining the final vote on an issue.

Parliamentarian	Each chamber has several parliamentarians who assist the presiding officer in several ways — interpreting the parliamentary rules under which that chamber operates, making rulings, and conducting the business of the chamber.
Pocket Veto	An action whereby the president withholds his or her approval of a bill and thereby vetoes it, after Congress has adjourned either for the year or for a specific period. When Congress is in session, a bill becomes law without the president's signature, if he or she does not act on it within ten days, excluding Sundays, from the time he or she receives it. However, if Congress adjourns within that ten-day period, the bill is killed without any formal veto action by the president.
Point of Order	A device to stop any pending business in the House to: 1) force a quorum call; 2) knock out bill language that does not pertain to the purpose of the bill; or 3) remove from the written record certain words spoken in violation of the House rules (e.g., name-calling, criticizing another Member personally).
President of the Senate	The vice president presides over the Senate. In his or her absence, a *president pro tempore* (Latin meaning, "president for the time being") presides.
President Pro Tempore	The chief officer of the Senate in the absence of the vice president. Elected by the other senators, he or she usually is the majority party senator with the longest continuous service in the Senate.
Private Calendar	In the House, private bills dealing with individual matters (e.g., claims against the government, immigration and naturalization) are put on this calendar.
Public Law (P.L.)	A measure that has passed both houses of Congress and been signed into law by the president. Laws are listed numerically by Congress. For example, Public Law 102-10 indicates that the bill was passed by the 102nd Congress and was the tenth measure passed by that Congress that was signed into law. Often abbreviated as *P.L.*
Quorum	The number of Members whose presence is necessary for the transaction of business. In the Senate and House, it is a majority of the membership (when there are no vacancies, this is 51 in the Senate and 218 in the House). A quorum is 100 in the Committee of the Whole House on the State of the Union. If a point of order is made that a quorum is not present, the only business in order is either a motion to adjourn or a motion to direct the sergeant-at-arms to request the attendance of absentee Members.
Recommit a Bill	A motion made on the floor, after deliberations on a bill and just before the final vote, to return that bill to the committee that reported it. Recommittal usually is considered a death blow. A motion to recommit may include instructions to the committee to report the bill again with specific amendments or by a certain date. The instructions may also be to conduct a particular study, with no definite deadline for final action.

Reconciliation	The 1974 Budget Act provides for a "reconciliation" procedure to bring tax and appropriations bills into conformity with congressional budget resolutions. Legislative committees must adjust revenues and expenditures by a certain amount and by a certain time. These recommendations are incorporated into one omnibus reconciliation bill which must then be approved by both houses of Congress.
Recorded Vote	A vote in which each Member's vote on a legislative proposal is recorded, either electronically or by a written tally.
Report	As a congressional term, both a verb and a noun. A committee, which has been examining a bill referred to it, *reports* its findings and recommendations to the chamber when the committee sends the bill to the chamber for consideration and a vote. This process is called *reporting* a bill. A *report* is the document setting forth the committee's explanation of its action on a bill. The report is sent to the chamber along with the bill. House and Senate reports are numbered separately and are designated as S. Rept. or H. Rept. Conference reports are numbered and designated in the same way as regular committee reports. Most reports favor a bill's passage, though there are often minority dissents from this majority position.
Resolution	A measure with no force of law (designated as S. Res. or H. Res.), passed only by the chamber in which it was introduced, and dealing only with business pertaining to that chamber. It does not require passage by the other chamber or approval by the president.
Rider	A measure unrelated to a bill but attached to it. A rider is used because the measure's sponsor hopes to get it through the legislative process more easily by attaching it to another piece of legislation instead of introducing it as a separate bill.
Roll Call	In either chamber, the clerk's calling the names of Members, either for the purpose of determining whether or not a quorum is present, or for taking a vote.
Rule	This term has two congressional meanings. A rule may be a standing order governing the conduct of House or Senate business and listed in the chamber's book of rules. The rules deal with matters including the duties of officers, order of business, attendance on the floor, and voting procedures. In the House, a rule also may be the procedure established by the House Rules Committee for floor debate on a particular bill.
Secretary of the Senate	Chief administrative officer of the Senate; responsible for directing the work of Senate employees, education of pages, administration of oaths of office, receipt of registration of lobbyists, and other activities necessary for the Senate's continuing administrative operation.
Select or Special Committee	A committee set up for a special purpose and a limited time by resolution of either the House or Senate. Most special committees are investigative in nature and have no legislative authority.

Sequestration	The automatic withholding of budgeted funds to keep the federal budget on target with deficit-reduction guidelines in a given fiscal year.
Slip Laws	The first official publication of a bill that has been signed into law. Each is published separately in unbound, single-sheet, or pamphlet form. It usually takes two to three days from the date of presidential signature to the time when slip laws become available.
Speaker	The presiding officer of the House of Representatives, elected from the majority party membership and by vote of that membership at the beginning of each new Congress.
Special Session	A session of Congress convened after it has adjourned *sine die*, completing its regular session. Special sessions are convened by the president under his constitutional powers (e.g., to declare war).
Standing Committees	The committees established permanently by House and Senate rules (see *Select* or *Special Committees*).
Supplemental Appropriations	An appropriations bill considered after passage of regular (annual) appropriations bills, and providing additional money for a government program during the course of a fiscal year. Requested by the executive branch, a supplemental appropriation is used to meet funding needs that were not anticipated during the regular appropriations process.
Suspension of the Rules	On the first and third Mondays of each month, and the last six days of a session, the Speaker of the House may entertain a motion to suspend the rules on legislation that is non-controversial. Under this procedure, debate is limited to twenty minutes on each side, no amendments are permitted, and the bill requires a two-thirds vote for passage.
Table	A motion used in both chambers to kill a bill, without having to vote on it directly. A motion to table cannot be debated and comes to an immediate vote. Once a bill is tabled, it is dead.
Teller Vote	Used in the House, but not in the Senate, to record total *yeas* and total *nays* and not how Members voted individually.
Tuesday Luncheons	In the Senate, each party holds a luncheon caucus for its Members each Tuesday. These sessions are used to plan the party's legislative strategy for the coming week and are seen as an integral part of Senate activity.
Unanimous Consent	Used in lieu of a vote on non-controversial motions, amendments, or bills. An objection by one Member will prevent consideration by unanimous consent.
Union Calendar	A House calendar containing bills that directly or indirectly appropriate money or raise revenue.
United States Code	A consolidation and codification of the general and permanent laws of the United States, arranged by subject matter under fifty titles. The code is revised periodically. Sample citation: 42 U.S.C. 1396d(a).

Veto	An action by the president rejecting a bill passed by Congress. When Congress is in session, the president must veto a bill within ten days of receiving it, excluding Sundays; otherwise, the bill becomes law without the president's signature. When the president vetoes a bill, it must be returned to the house of origin with a *veto message* stating the president's objections. A presidential veto may be overridden by a two-thirds vote of the membership in the House and in the Senate (see *Override*).
Views and Estimates	Reports prepared by House and Senate standing committees presenting their views on the presidential budget requests, for a given fiscal year, that are within their purviews. These are submitted by the standing committees to the budget committees to assist in developing the budget resolution.
Voice Vote	In either the House or Senate, members answer "aye" or "no" in chorus and the presiding officer decides which group has more votes. Often followed by a recorded vote on the same measure.
Well	The area in front of the Speaker's rostrum in the House from which Members may address the House. Senators speak from their desks.
Whip	See *Majority Whip, Minority Whip*.
Without Objection	Used in lieu of a vote on non-controversial motions, amendments, or bills, an order from the chairman/chairwoman which allows a measure to be approved in either the House or the Senate if no Member voices an objection.
Yielding	When a Member has been recognized to speak, no other Member may speak without permission from the Member recognized by the chairman/chairwoman. This permission is called *yielding* and usually is requested in the form, "Will the gentleman/gentlelady yield?"

GLOSSARY OF MEDIA TERMS

Actuality brief on-scene report, live or taped, for radio news broadcast.

Angle the emphasis or approach of a news story.

Backgrounder document covering relevant facts and significance of issue or event; provides information basic to understanding of issue or event.

Bite sound bite; five- to ten-second portion of an interviewee's comments, used in radio or television news or feature story.

Edit Memo A memorandum to an editorial page editor requesting a meeting or an editorial on a specific issue or event.

Fact Sheet an advisory information sheet designed to generate on-scene media coverage of an event.

Media Alert A one-page announcement of an event of interest to the media (a press conference, press opportunity).

News Kit A packet of material which supplies all the background information a reporter needs on an issue to write a story (do not overdo it).

Pitch Letter A personalized letter requesting coverage of an issue or event and an explanation as to why it is newsworthy.

Public Service Announcement (PSA) A written announcement — in formats of twenty, thirty, or sixty seconds — used by radio and television stations to fill gaps between programming and paid advertising. PSAs cannot be partisan or support or oppose legislation. They alert people to meetings and provide information.

Release Date Time and date on which information issued to the media may be released to the public. The media is under no legal responsibility to honor release date or embargoes.

Sidebar Secondary story that accompanies main news story or feature article.

Slug Line Words placed at upper left corner of second and subsequent pages of news release or news story for identification purposes.

Style Book Manual of standards for copywriting.

Tabloid Newspaper format, smaller than standard size, usually five-column.

Trade publications Periodicals covering issues of interest to a specific industry, profession, or occupation.

ACRONYMS IN THE HEALTH CARE INDUSTRY

WHO'S WHO AND WHAT'S WHAT IN THE WASHINGTON, DC HEALTH CARE INDUSTRY

When one is dealing with contacts in Washington, DC, it becomes apparent that people in the nation's capital speak a different language. Whether you are talking with someone in Congress, in a federal agency, or in the health care industry, you probably will have to decipher certain codes to understand the everyday language of Washington bureaucrats and operatives. To give you a head start, a partial list of "Washington acronyms" connected to the health care industry is presented below.

AACN	American Association of Critical Care Nurses
AACN	American Association of Colleges of Nursing
AAHA	American Association of Homes for the Aging
AAHE	Association for the Advancement of Health Education
AANA	American Association of Nurse Anesthetists
AANN	American Association of Neuroscience Nurses
AAOHN	American Association of Occupational Health Nurses
AARP	American Association of Retired Persons
AART	American Association for Respiratory Therapy
AASCIN	American Association of Spinal Cord Injury Nurses
AAUW	American Association of University Women
ABC	American Blood Commission
ACCMRTS	American Certification Council of Medical Rehabilitation Therapists and Specialists
ACHA	American College of Hospital Administrators
ACIL	American Council of Independent Laboratories
ACLA	American Clinical Laboratory Association
ACNHA	American College of Nursing Home Administrators
ACNM	American College of Nurse Midwives

ACS	American Chemical Society
ADA	American Dental Association
AFGE	American Federation of Government Employees
AFSCME	American Federation of State, County, and Municipal Employees
AFL-CIO	American Federation of Labor-Congress of Industrial Organizations
AHA	American Hospital Association
AHCA	American Health Care Association
AHCPR	Agency for Health Care Policy and Research (HHS)
AIDS	Acquired Immune Deficiency Syndrome
AMA	American Medical Association
ANA	American Nurses Association
ANNA	American Nephrology Nurses Association
AOA	American Osteopathic Association
AORN	Association of Operating Room Nurses
APA	American Psychiatric Association
APA	American Psychological Association
APHA	American Public Health Association
APIC	Association for Practitioners in Infection Control
APON	Association of Pediatric Oncology Nurses
ARN	Association of Rehabilitation Nurses
ASAHP	American Society of Allied Health Professions
ASHP	American Society of Hospital Pharmacists
ASORN	American Society of Ophthalmic Registered Nurses
ASPAN	American Society of Post Anesthesia Nurses
ASPRSN	American Society of Plastic and Reconstructive Surgical Nurses, Inc.
AWHONN	Association of Women's Health, Obstetric, and Neonatal Nurses
BLS	Bureau of Labor Statistics (DOL)
BPW	National Federation of Business and Professional Women
CBO	Congressional Budget Office
CDC	Centers for Disease Control
CGFNS	Commission on Graduate Foreign Nursing Schools
CNM	Certified Nurse Midwife
CNO	Community Nursing Organization
CNS	Clinical Nurse Specialist

CRS	Congressional Research Service (Library of Congress)
DNC	Democratic National Committee
DOD	Department of Defense
DOL	Department of Labor
DVA	Department of Veterans' Affairs
EBRI	Employee Benefits Research Institute
ENA	Emergency Nurses Association
EPA	Environmental Protection Agency
ERTA	Economic Recovery Tax Act
FAH	Federation of American Hospitals
FDA	Food and Drug Administration (HHS)
FEC	Federal Election Commission
FEHPB	Federal Employees Health Benefits Program
FTC	Federal Trade Commission
FY	Fiscal Year
GAO	General Accounting Office
GPO	Government Printing Office
HBV	Hepatitis B Virus
HCFA	Health Care Financing Administration (HHS)
HHS	Department of Health and Human Services
HIAA	Health Insurance Association of America
HIV	Human Immunodeficiency Virus
HMO	Health Maintenance Organization
IAET	International Association for Enterostomal Therapy, Inc.
IHS	Indian Health Service
IOM	Institute of Medicine
JCAH	Joint Commission on the Accreditation of Hospitals
JCAHO	Joint Commission on the Accreditation of Health Care Organizations
LPN	Licensed Practical Nurse
LVN	Licensed Vocational Nurse
NAM	National Association of Manufacturers
NAON	National Association of Orthopedic Nurses
NAPH	National Association of Public Hospitals

NAPNAP	National Association of Pediatric Nurse Associates and Practitioners
NANPRH	National Association of Nurse Practitioners in Reproductive Health
NASN	National Association of School Nurses
NASW	National Association of Social Workers
NAPM	National Association of Pharmaceutical Manufacturers
NBNA	National Black Nurses Association
NCNR	National Center for Nursing Research
NEA	Nurse Education Act
NFNA	National Flight Nurses Association
NIH	National Institutes of Health (HHS)
NIMH	National Institutes of Mental Health (HHS)
NIOSH	National Institute of Occupational Safety and Health (DOL)
NLRA	National Labor Relations Act
NLRB	National Labor Relations Board
NNSA	National Nurses' Society on Addiction
NOW	National Organization for Women
NP	Nurse Practitioner
OBRA	Omnibus Budget Reconciliation Act
OMB	Office of Management and Budget
ONS	Oncology Nurses Society
OPM	Office of Personnel Management
OSHA	Occupational Safety and Health Administration (DOL)
OTA	Office of Technology Assessment
PAC	Political Action Committee
PHS	Public Health Service (HHS)
PMA	Pharmaceutical Manufacturers Association
PPO	Preferred Provider Organization
PPRC	Physician Payment Review Commission
PRO	Peer Review Organization
PROPAC	Prospective Payment Assessment Commission
PSRO	Professional Standards Review Organization
RN	Registered Nurse

RNC	Republican National Committee
SEIU	Service Employees International Union
SNF	Skilled Nursing Facility
TAANA	The American Association of Nurse Attorneys
TEFRA	Tax Equity and Fiscal Responsibility Act
UR	Utilization Review
VNA	Visiting Nurses Association
WREI	Women's Research Education Institute

KEY OFFICES/OFFICIALS
OF THE FEDERAL AGENCIES

THE WHITE HOUSE

The White House
1600 Pennsylvania Avenue, NW
Washington, DC 20500
(202) 456-1414

- Office of the President
  (202) 456-2168

- Office of the Vice President
  (202) 456-2326

- Office of the Chief of Staff
  (202) 456-6797

- Office of the First Lady
  (202) 456-2957

- Office of the Press Secretary
  (202) 456-2100

- Counsel to the President
  (202) 456-2632

- Presidential Appointments/
  Scheduling
  (202) 456-2825

- Presidential Personnel Office
  (202) 456-7060

- Office of Bill Clerk
  (202) 456-2226

- Office of Legislative Affairs
  (202) 456-2230

- Office of Political Affairs
  (202) 456-2135

- Office of Public Liaison
  (202) 456-7900

OFFICE OF THE PRESIDENT

Office of Management and Budget
Old Executive Office Building
17th Street and Pennsylvania Ave., NW
Washington, DC 20503

- Director
  (202) 395-4840

Office of National Drug Control Policy
Executive Office of the President
Washington, DC 20500

- Director
  (202) 467-9800

CABINET-LEVEL FEDERAL AGENCIES

Department of Agriculture
14th Street and Independence Ave., SW
Washington, DC 20250
(202) 447-3631

Department of Commerce
15th Street and Constitution Ave., NW
Washington, DC 20230
(202) 377-2112

Department of Defense
The Pentagon
Washington, DC 20301
(703) 695-5261

- Assistant Secretary, Health Affairs
  (703) 697-2111

- Department of the Air Force
  Chief, Air Force Nurse Corps
  (202) 767-5074

- Department of the Army
  Chief, Army Nurse Corps
  (703) 756-0045

- Department of the Navy
  Director, Navy Nurse Corps
  (202) 653-0124

Department of Education
400 Maryland Ave., SW
Washington, DC 20202
(202) 401-3000

Department of Energy
1000 Independence Ave., SW
Washington, DC 20585
(202) 586-6210

Department of Health and Human Services
200 Independence Ave., SW
Washington, DC 20201
(202) 245-7000

- Assistant Secretary, Health
  (202) 245-7694

- Assistant Secretary, Administration
  for Children and Families
  (202) 401-9200

- Assistant Secretary, Legislation
  (202) 245-7627

- Health Care Financing
  Administration
  200 Independence Ave., SW
  Washington, DC 20201
  (202) 245-6726

- Office of Legislation and Policy
  (202) 426-3960

- Medicaid Bureau
  (301) 966-3870

- **Public Health Service**

  > Surgeon General
    (301) 245-6467

  > Deputy Surgeon General
    (301) 443-4000

  > Agency for Health Care Policy
    and Research
    (301) 443-5650

  > Centers for Disease Control
    (404) 639-3291

  > Food and Drug Administration
    (301) 443-2410

  > Health Resources and Services
    Administration
    (301) 443-2216

  > National Health Service Corps
    (301) 443-2900

  > Nursing Division
    (301) 443-5786

  > Indian Health Services
    (301) 443-1083

  > National Institutes of Health
    (301) 496-2433

  > National Center For Nursing
    Research
    (301) 496-0523

**Department of Housing and
Urban Development**
451 7th St., SW
Washington, DC 20410
(202) 708-0417

Department of the Interior
18th and C Streets, NW
Washington, DC 20240
(202) 208-7351

- Assistant Secretary, Indian Affairs
  (202) 208-7163

Department of Justice
Constitution Ave. and 10th St., NW
Washington, DC 20530
(202) 514-2101

Department of Labor
200 Constitution Ave., NW
Washington, DC 20210
(202) 523-8271

- Occupational Safety and Health
  Administration
  (202) 523-7162

Department of State
2201 C St., NW
Washington, DC 20520
(202) 647-4910

Department of Transportation
400 7th St., SW
Washington, DC 20590
(202) 366-1111

Department of the Treasury
15th St. and Pennsylvania Ave., NW
Washington, DC 20220
(202) 566-2533

Department of Veterans' Affairs
810 Vermont Ave., NW
Washington, DC 20420
(202) 233-3775

- Deputy Assistant Chief Medical
  Director for Nursing Programs
  (202) 535-7364

RELATED FEDERAL AGENCIES

Internal Revenue Service
1111 Constitution Ave., NW
Washington, DC 20224
(202) 566-4743

Office of Personnel Management
1900 E Street, NW
Washington, DC 20415
(202) 606-1000

National Labor Relations Board
1717 Pennsylvania Ave., NW
Washington, DC 20570
(202) 254-8064

SUPREME COURT

Supreme Court Building
1 First St., NE
Washington, DC 20543
(202) 479-3000

- Administrative Assistant to
  the Chief Justice
  (202) 479-3400

- Clerk
  (202) 479-3014

- Public Information
  (202) 479-3211

KEY POLITICAL CONTACTS

Federal Election Commission
999 E St., NW
Washington, DC 20463
(202) 219-4104
(202) 219-4134

Democratic National Committee
430 South Capitol St., SE
Washington, DC 20003
(202) 863-8000

Republican National Committee
310 First St., SE
Washington, DC 20003
(202) 863-8500

KEY MEDIA CONTACTS

American Broadcasting Company (ABC)
1717 De Sales St., NW
Washington, DC 20036
Bureau Chief   (202) 887-7777

Columbia Broadcasting System (CBS)
2020 M St., NW
Washington, DC 20036
Bureau Chief   (202) 457-4321

National Broadcasting Company (NBC)
4001 Nebraska Ave., NW
Washington, DC 20016
Bureau Chief   (202) 885-4000

Cable News Network (CNN)
820 First St., NE, #1100
Washington, DC 20002
Bureau Chief   (202) 898-7900

United Press International (UPI)
1400 Eye St., NW, #800
Washington, DC 20005
Bureau Chief   (202) 898-7000

Associated Press (AP)
2021 K St., NW , #600
Washington, DC 20006
Bureau Chief   (202) 828-6432

KEY LEGISLATIVE CONTACTS

SENATE LEADERSHIP

Majority Leader	(202) 224-5556
Majority Whip	(202) 224-2158
Minority Leader	(202) 224-3135
Minority Whip	(202) 224-2708

Senate Telephone Directory

Bill Clerk	(202) 224-2120
Cloakroom, Democratic	(202) 224-4691
Cloakroom, Republican	(202) 224-6391
Document Room	(202) 224-7860
Legislative Counsel	(202) 224-6461
Periodical Press Gallery	(202) 224-0265
Press Gallery	(202) 224-0241
Radio and Television Gallery	(202) 224-6421

HOUSE LEADERSHIP

Speaker	(202) 225-5604
Majority Leader	(202) 225-0100
Majority Whip	(202) 225-3130
Minority Leader	(202) 225-0600
Minority Whip	(202) 225-2800

House of Representatives Telephone Directory

Bill Status	(202) 225-1772
Chief Bill Clerk	(202) 225-7925
Clerk of the House	(202) 225-7000
Cloakroom, Democratic	(202) 225-7330
Cloakroom, Republican	(202) 225-7350
Document Room	(202) 225-3456
LEGIS (Legislative Info. System)	(202) 225-1772
Periodical Press Gallery	(202) 225-2941
Press Gallery	(202) 225-3945
Radio and Television Gallery	(202) 225-5214

MISCELLANEOUS CAPITOL HILL OFFICES

Congressional Black Caucus	(202) 226-7790
Congressional Caucus for Women's Issues	(202) 225-6740
Congressional Hispanic Caucus	(202) 226-3430
Congressional Budget Office	(202) 226-2600
Congressional Research Service	(202) 707-5775
Democratic Congressional Campaign Committee	(202) 863-1500
Democratic Senatorial Campaign Committee	(202) 224-2447
House Democratic Caucus	(202) 226-3210
House Republican Conference	(202) 225-5107
Library of Congress	(202) 707-2905
National Republican Congressional Committee	(202) 479-7000
National Republican Senatorial Committee	(202) 675-6000
Office of Technology Assessment	(202) 224-3695
Senate Democratic Policy Committee	(202) 224-5551
Senate Republican Policy Committee	(202) 224-2946

MISCELLANEOUS GENERAL NUMBERS

Capitol Switchboard

Senate	(202) 224-3121
House	(202) 225-3121

Congressional Record Index   (202) 275-9009

General Accounting Office
Documents Distribution   (202) 275-6241

Government Printing Office
Order Desk   (202) 783-3238

Federal Register, Statutes Unit

(public law numbers, statutory
references, presidential
proclamations)   (202) 523-5230

Public Laws Update Services
(a recording about public laws
signed too recently for inclusion
by statutes unit)   (202) 523-6641

Library of Congress

Congressional Research Service   (202) 707-5700

Copyright Application Forms
Requests   (202) 707-9100

Copyright Information   (202) 479-0700

Photo-Duplication Service

(Information on duplicating
materials available in the
collection of the library)   (202) 707-5640

Telephone Reference Assistance   (202) 707-5522

"EVEN IF YOU'RE ON THE RIGHT TRACK,
YOU CAN GET RUN OVER IF YOU'RE
JUST SITTING THERE."

Will Rogers
American humorist

WHEN IT'S CRUCIAL TO KEEP UP WITH NEWS AT THE FEDERAL LEVEL...

IT'S TIME FOR *CAPITAL UPDATE*!

The only comprehensive newsletter for nurses containing:

➡ **LEGISLATIVE UPDATES**

➡ **CAMPAIGN AND OTHER POLITICAL INFORMATION**

➡ **FEDERAL AGENCY REGULATORY DEVELOPMENTS**

When you subscribe to *Capital Update*, you'll have personal access to ANA's careful, concise and condensed analyses of nursing issues at the federal level. You'll also be informed about ANA's activities in relation to your concerns...concerns such as workplace advocacy, health care reform, family and medical leave, activities of Senate and House health committees, AIDS, Medicare and Medicaid, OSHA regulations, maternal and child health, rural health, and more.

Decisions that affect the profession of nursing and the delivery of health care are made every day in Washington, DC. *Capital Update* not only reports on these issues, but explains how these issues affect you, the individual nurse. The best part — *Capital Update* is a real bargain. No other publication gives you so much information — eight pages full of critical legislative and regulatory news — so often — 24 times a year — and at such an affordable price. If you subscribe to *Capital Update* now, you may purchase one copy of *The Grassroots Lobbying Handbook: Empowering Nurses through Legislative and Political Action* at a 15-percent discount (i.e., SNA member price, $17.00; non-member price, $25.50).

➡ Send your check or money order with a note requesting *Capital Update* to:

> *Capital Update*
> Subscriptions
> Accounting Department
> American Nurses Association
> 600 Maryland Avenue, SW
> Suite 100 West
> Washington, DC 20024-2571

➡ If you are interested in receiving *The Grassroots Lobbying Handbook* at a 15- percent discount with your subscription to *Capital Update*, send your *separate* check or money order *for the Handbook* with a note referring to **SPECIAL OFFER GR-00** to

> American Nurses Publishing
> Distribution Center,
> P.O. Box 4100
> Kearneysville, WV 25430.

INTERESTED? SUBSCRIPTION RATES ARE:

❏ **$25 ANA COUNCIL AFFILIATE (Provide name of Council)**

❏ **$25 STUDENT RATE (Provide name of school)**

❏ **$50 SNA MEMBER (Provide SNA membership #)**

❏ **$75 NON-MEMBER**

❏ **$100 INSTITUTIONAL RATE**